# Policing sexual assault

Since the 1970s, feminist campaigners have put pressure on govern-
ments to take the issue of male violence seriously. By focusing on
research in Britain and other countries, *Policing Sexual Assault* traces
the ways in which the criminal justice system has responded to feminist
demands for improvements in service and access to justice for the
victims of domestic and sexual violence. It includes the first survey of
police recording practices of male rape and also presents a detailed
account of the experiences of women complainants, their views of the
police, the medical examination and court procedures. The link is
made between the treatment of complainants and internal policies on
the recruitment and promotion of women officers and the growing
scandal of sexual harassment within the force. Also assessed are the
role of the Crown Prosecution Service and factors associated with the
dramatic fall in the conviction rate for rape.

*Policing Sexual Assault* draws on original research and other studies
to develop insights into policing violence and presents the case for
radical reform.

**Jeanne Gregory** is Visiting Professor and Head of the Gender Research
Centre, Middlesex University.

**Sue Lees** is Professor of Women's Studies and Director of the Centre
for Research in Ethnicity and Gender, University of North London.

# Policing sexual assault

**Jeanne Gregory and Sue Lees**

London and New York

First published 1999
by Routledge
11 New Fetter Lane, London EC4P 4EE

Simultaneously published in the USA and Canada
by Routledge
29 West 35th Street, New York, NY 10001

© 1999 Jeanne Gregory and Sue Lees

Typeset in Times by Routledge
Printed and bound in Great Britain by
Creative Print and Design (Wales), Ebbw Vale

*British Library Cataloguing in Publication Data*
A catalogue record for this book is available from the British Library

*Library of Congress Cataloging in Publication Data*
Gregory, Jeanne.
  Policing sexual assault / Jeanne Gregory and Sue Lees.
  Includes bibliographical references and index.
  1. Rape–Investigation–Great Britain. 2. Women–Crimes against–
  Great Britain. 3. Sex discrimination in criminal justice
  administration–Great Britain. I. Lees, Sue. II. Title.
HV8079.R35G74  1998                         98–8111
364.15`32`0941–dc21                         CIP


ISBN  0–415–16387–0 (hbk)
ISBN  0–415–16388–9 (pbk)

# Contents

# Tables

# Acknowledgements

We would like to thank Trevor Jones and Michael Pollak of Islington Council Police Support Committee and Crime Prevention Unit for making the research possible. We would particularly like to thank the two policewomen who collected some of the data for us, and other police officers who agreed to be interviewed. Many others provided us with information, advice and support during the research, including Robin Allen QC, Jennifer Brown, Lynn Ferguson, Debbie King, Tina Martin, Phil Rumney and Jennifer Temkin. We would also like to thank Sue Sharpe for conducting some of the interviews. Most of all we appreciate the participation of all the women who were prepared to relive their experiences.

# 1 Introduction

During the 1980s and 1990s there has been a sea change in the recognition of male violence against women and children, not only in Britain, but in many other parts of the world. In the 1970s women in North America, Australia and Britain set up crisis centres and refuges where women could escape from violence by their partners, husbands or fathers. Feminists began a long-running campaign to give women more protection from the police, the courts and the law. By the 1990s, important changes in police practices and a changed climate of opinion had encouraged an increasing number of women to report violence to the police. Policies on sexual harassment were developed by employers in both the public and private sectors and the last decade has seen a developing awareness on this issue and a proliferation of 'good practice' guidelines. This book charts some of these developments in relation to sexual assault on women (and some men), but reveals that we are still a long way from achieving what the Labour Party consultation document (1995) optimistically referred to as the elimination of domestic and sexual violence. Police practice is a crucial barometer of both the advances and limits of progress in this field.

The issue of violence against women is now on the agenda at an international level, both in the United Nations and the Council of Europe. In July 1997 UNICEF included in its annual Progress of Nations report a specific section on violence against women where progress is defined according to the degree of protection women have against discrimination and violence. In 1986 the European Parliament endorsed a wide-ranging report submitted by its Women's Committee on all aspects of violence against women (European Parliament 1986). The report included a number of recommendations concerning police practices: first, that police officers should be trained to deal with victims in a sympathetic, constructive and reassuring manner; second, that the police should inform the victim of the possibilities of obtaining assistance, practical and legal advice, compensation from the offender and from the state; third, that the victim should be able to obtain information on the outcome of the police investigation (Joutsen 1987).

In 1994 the General Assembly of the Organization of American States adopted an Inter-American Convention on the Prevention, Punishment and Eradication of Violence against Women and the Inter-American Development Bank has a project on the cost of violence against women. On a global level, the World Bank includes in its annual assessment of Gross National Product working time lost due to violence against women. The United Nations Declaration on the Elimination of Violence against Women was adopted in 1993 and the Declaration and Platform for Action at the UN Fourth World Conference on Women in Beijing in 1995 included 'violence' as one of twelve 'critical areas of concern' impeding women's advancement. As Rosalind Coward pointed out (*Guardian*, 24 July 1997), the feminist rhetoric being used is staggeringly bold. There is a new category of 'gender crime' to refer to such practices as bride burning,[1] domestic beatings and genital mutilation, which have previously been seen as isolated phenomena rather than acknowledged as the results of patriarchal dominance.

Child abuse has become an issue of public concern and a key media issue (see Skidmore 1995). UNICEF calculates that trafficking in children is the third most lucrative illegal trade in the world, after drugs and weapons, and is a multi-billion dollar business. It is estimated that 5,000 children work in the sex trade in Britain and are the victims of family abuse, career paedophiles, prostitution, sex tourism and pornography. It is also estimated that there are 30,000 paedophiles organized in groups throughout Europe linked through the Internet and on the mailing lists of pornographic magazines. In Belgium, the arrest of a paedophile gang, who had abducted teenage girls and allowed two 8 year olds to starve to death in an underground prison, led to suspicion of police involvement in the atrocities (see Bates 1996).

This book investigates the impact of a recent concerted effort in Britain to change the way in which women (and more recently, men) reporting sexual attacks are dealt with by the front line agents for the criminal justice system, the police. It is one of the first studies of the reporting of sexual assault since the creation of the Crown Prosecution Service (CPS) in England and Wales in 1986. The CPS assumed the main responsibility for the prosecution of criminal cases, a task formerly undertaken by the police. (In Scotland there has always been an independent prosecutor, the Procurator Fiscal.) The change coincides with a steady fall in the conviction rate for rape and attempted rape in England and Wales from 24 per cent of reported cases in 1985 to 10 per cent in 1996 (Home Office Statistics). The arrest rate for cases of domestic violence remains at 14 per cent with even fewer cases proceeding to prosecution (Labour Party 1995). Unfortunately research into the prosecution process and into court procedures and sentencing practices in cases involving male violence is sparse.

There is, however, a growing body of research on the issue of police responses to domestic violence and sexual assault (see Faragher 1985, Edwards 1989, Bourlet 1990, Mullender 1996, Temkin 1997a). It is clear that the police have a crucial role to play in any attempt to implement a strategy designed to close the gap between the official condemnation of male violence as enshrined in the law and the realities of male violence as condoned in practice. Yet at the same time the police reflect the status quo; predominantly white, male and conservative in outlook; they are themselves part of a macho culture which is profoundly anti-feminist. Any attempts to introduce radical changes in the way in which cases of male violence are handled by the police must therefore confront two major obstacles: the first is the 'enemy within', i.e. resistance from police culture; the second is the 'enemy without', which is the refusal of the other major players in the criminal justice system, from the Crown Prosecution Service to the Court of Appeal, to accept that a fundamentally new approach to the problem of male violence is needed.

## Police forces under attack

Police forces in England and Wales have found themselves under severe attack in recent years from a number of different quarters. They stand accused of racism in their dealings with black and minority ethnic communities and of sexism in their dealings with women, particularly those reporting crimes involving male violence. Additionally, they have been subjected to a range of criticisms which, when considered together, appear to be making contradictory demands on them. On the one hand, falling rates of detection and conviction across a range of serious crimes give rise to the belief that crime is spiralling out of police control; on the other hand, there is incontrovertible evidence that the police are prepared to take short cuts in order to secure a conviction, particularly where public outrage demands a quick result. The long-running investigation into the techniques used by the West Midlands Serious Crime Squad to obtain confessions has seriously shaken public confidence in the integrity of the police service. The most spectacular miscarriages of justice, such as the Guildford Four, the Birmingham Six, the Maguire Seven, the Broadwater Farm Three and the Bridgewater Three sent shock waves reverberating throughout the criminal justice system (Rose 1996a).

In relation to rape and sexual assault, the police stand accused of employing harsh methods of interrogation on women reporting such attacks, on the assumption that they might be making false allegations. In 1982, the Thames Valley Police Force was pleased to allow such an interrogation to be shown on BBC television as part of a documentary series on police work, confident that their professionalism would be applauded. They were completely taken aback by the public outcry that followed, with the *Guardian* describing the interview as a display of 'unmitigated toughness' and 'low-key brutality' (quoted in Scott and Dickens 1989). This single incident provided the impetus to reform the procedures by which violence against women is policed, at a time of rapidly changing attitudes towards the treatment of women. The rediscovery of child sexual abuse in Cleveland and the subsequent furore resulted in a re-examination of children's experiences of the criminal justice system.

However, as Radford and Stanko point out (1996) the changes are likely to have more to do with the influences of North American police practices in managing inner-city riots than with a desire to combat violence against women and children. They argue that in shifting the focus to crime against women, the police were adopting the mantle of protectors of women and children and attempting to 'renegotiate some consensus in the inner city' (ibid. 70, see also Sim *et al.* 1987). Radford and Stanko review attempts by North American feminists to take class action law suits against entire police forces so that failure to take action can cost the police dearly (Ferraro 1989).

In later chapters we present the findings of our own research, designed to contribute to this process of analysis and policy formation. Here we give an account of some of the earlier studies which turned the spotlight on police policies and practices in relation to crimes of male violence.

## Improving service delivery

The Metropolitan Police took the criticisms of the investigation techniques, as demonstrated by the Thames Valley Police, very much to heart and put in train a series of measures designed to improve service delivery to women reporting rape and sexual assault. A 1983 Home Office circular (25/83) issued to chief constables was designed to ensure that women reporting sexual attacks would be treated with tact and sympathy and in 1984 the Women's National Commission (WNC) established a working group on violence against women in order to monitor these developments and to make further recommendations for change. Their report *Violence Against Women* (WNC 1985) showed that police forces across England and Wales were beginning to respond to the new policy guidelines but that much remained to be done, particularly with regard to police training. Another major area of concern was the shortage of women police officers to conduct interviews with complainants and of women doctors to undertake medical examinations, despite the expressed preference of many complainants for their cases to be dealt with by women professionals.

In relation to domestic violence, the report revealed that police officers were frequently reluctant to intervene in domestic disputes or did so in a judgmental way, often siding with the man. The need for training was again emphasized, together with a recommendation that the law be changed to ensure that rape within marriage was regarded as a crime in all circumstances. The report recommended that the Home Secretary issue a further circular, focusing particularly on the question of training. With the publication of the report came a commitment by the Metropolitan Police to make further improvements in relation to sexual assault cases, including training for detective inspectors to give them some understanding of rape trauma syndrome (see Chapter 6) and the establishment of rape examination suites where complainants could be medically examined in comfortable surroundings (Metropolitan Police press release, February 1985, reprinted in WNC 1985). These initiatives were reinforced by Home Office circular 69/86 which called for new police training inputs on rape and sexual assault, the appointment of more women officers and better facilities for medical examinations.

In collecting evidence for their report, the WNC focused exclusively on experiences and policy developments in England and Wales and yet some of the pioneering research on the issue of rape and sexual assault has occurred under the auspices of the Scottish Office. The path-breaking study by Chambers and Millar, *Investigating Sexual Assault*, was published in 1983. Based on interviews with 70 women reporting rape or sexual assault, the study found that the majority of complainants were critical of 'the unsympathetic and tactless manner' with which the police conducted their interviews (ibid. 94). The researchers pointed out that the skills 'appropriate for interrogating offenders are not appropriate for interviewing sexual assault complainers or other witnesses' (ibid. 131). The sceptical approach adopted by the police meant that complainants were often discouraged from telling their full story and would even elaborate or distort what actually happened in a desperate effort to be believed. This merely reinforced police scepticism and consolidated their view that women make false allegations. In emphasizing the need for police training in interviewing techniques, Chambers and Millar insist that the goals of apprehending the offender and of dealing sympathetically with complainants are not in conflict. On the contrary, a strategy of putting the complainant's well-being first and foremost would actually benefit the progress of the case and increase the likelihood of a successful outcome.

## Reporting sexual assault

A number of studies have indicated that the proportion of rapes reported is very low. A student union survey at Cambridge University in 1994 found that one in five of the 1,500 students questioned reported that they had been victims of rape or attempted rape and one in nine that they had been raped; only one in fifty had told the police (BBC 2 *Public Eye* 1992). Another student union survey of 2,000 women at Oxford Brookes University revealed that 90 per cent of women who had never been sexually assaulted thought that they would report it to the police, yet in fact only 6 per cent of those who had been attacked had in fact reported it. When women were asked why they did not report, they said they feared an unsympathetic response from the police and had little faith in the judicial system (Faizey 1994).

Liz Kelly, who undertook a detailed study of women's experiences of sexual violence, pointed out that for women to identify themselves as victims or survivors of sexual violence, they must first define what has happened to them as lying outside the normal, as abusive. In order to consider reporting it to the police, they would need themselves to perceive the behaviour as a crime. The sixty women who participated in her research were volunteers, most of whom came forward as a result of a series of talks on sexual violence she gave to a range of different women's groups. She asked them about their experiences of various forms of sexual violence, including threats of violence, sexual harassment, sexual assault, obscene telephone calls, flashing, domestic violence, rape and incest. The incidence ranged from 100 per cent in the case of threats of violence to 22 per cent in the case of incest. Overall, less than 1 per cent of the events documented during the research were reported to the police and only five men were charged with offences. Low levels of reporting and low levels of police action ranged across the entire spectrum of offences. For example, 76 incidents of flashing were recalled by 30 of the women; 4 of these incidents were reported and no man was charged with an offence. Twenty-eight of the women had been raped, 6 within marriage, and only 8 of these cases had been reported to the police. Half of these were dropped (including two marital rapes), two women withdrew their complaints after hours of interrogation and two cases went to court; neither woman was informed of the outcome (Kelly 1988, chapter 4).

These findings confirm that even when women did perceive male violence as a crime, they placed little reliance on the police to offer them effective protection. Similarly, in the *Violence Against Women – Women Speak Out* survey conducted in Wandsworth between September 1983 and August 1984, fewer than one-quarter of the incidents of male violence experienced by the 314 women who participated were reported to the police. The reasons for not reporting given most often were that the women believed the police were not interested in 'routine' sexual and racial harassment and that they could not or would not take action; or they expected the police to be unpleasant or unsympathetic (Radford 1987). The women in Kelly's survey had expressed very similar sentiments (Kelly 1988). There is some evidence that black women may be more likely to report domestic violence to the police. This could reflect a higher rate of victimization or could be due to other reasons (see Chapter 4).

## Recording sexual assault

The reluctance of many women to report sexual attacks to the police is compounded by the falling away of the majority of the cases that are reported at various stages in the criminal justice process, resulting in very low conviction rates.

It is impossible to know with any degree of certainty how many sexual attacks take place in Britain each year. Estimates vary according to the methodology employed: on the one hand, the British Crime Surveys, involving interviews with people in their own homes, uncover almost no reports of rape or sexual assault; on the other hand, a women's safety questionnaire, distributed to women in London at various public venues during the summer of 1982, found that of the women who responded, two in every five had experienced rape, attempted rape or another form of sexual assault at least once (Hall 1985). It could be argued that the methodology used, in sharp contrast to that used by the British Crime surveys, could lead to an overestimation of the incidence of rape, insofar as women who have been attacked may be more likely to respond (although many more may feel too traumatized to take part), but the findings in relation to the proportion of the women who subsequently reported the attack to the police are incontrovertible. Excluding the women who had been raped by their husbands (as this was in most cases not considered a crime in 1982), only 8 per cent of the women reporting rape to the researchers had reported it to the police; for sexual assaults, the figure was 18 per cent. When the women who had not reported to the police were asked to give reasons for this, 72 per cent replied that they believed the police would be unhelpful or unsympathetic; when women reporting rape were considered separately, this figure rose to 79 per cent (Hall 1985).

According to Home Office statistics, the number of cases of rape and sexual assault reported to the police in England and Wales has trebled during the last ten years. This may be due to an actual increase in the number of these crimes or to a greater willingness on the part of those who have been attacked to come forward, in the expectation that their complaint will be handled more sympathetically in the wake of the new policies and procedures. It may also be due in part to the new procedures themselves, particularly the tightening of the 'no criming' rules. This refers to the police practice of not recording some of the crimes reported to them, so that they never appear in the official statistics at all. According to earlier studies, levels of 'no criming' were particularly high in relation to reports of rape and sexual assault and astronomically high in cases of domestic violence.

In a study involving six English counties, Richard Wright found that 24 per cent of reports of rape and attempted rape were 'no crimed' (Wright 1984) and in the Scottish Office study, the 'no crime' figure was 22 per cent (Chambers and Millar 1983). The Metropolitan Police review of procedures sought to ensure that from 1985 allegations of rape and sexual assault would be 'no crimed' only when they were shown to be false or malicious. A Home Office study of two London Boroughs (Lambeth and Islington) was able to measure the impact of this policy change by examining the attrition between reporting and recording in 1984 and in 1986 (Smith 1989a). The levels of 'no criming' revealed in this study were extremely high, but there was a marked decline during the two year period, so that the proportion of cases 'no crimed' fell from 61 per cent in 1984 to 38 per cent in 1986. The apparent increase in rape during this period was entirely due to the changes in recording practice, as the number of rapes reported actually fell slightly during the two years. Even so, the researchers found a number of cases 'no crimed' on the basis of the woman withdrawing her complaint, although there was no evidence that the allegation had been false. In other words, police officers were still not complying fully with the advice given (Smith 1989a).

A nationwide Home Office study conducted in the second quarter of 1985 found that a quarter of the cases were 'no crimed' (Grace *et al.* 1992). However, the sample excluded cases 'no crimed' during the first month after the date of reporting and so underestimated the extent of 'no criming'. The different methodologies employed and the different geographical coverage of these various studies make direct comparison difficult, but it seems clear that by the mid 1980s 'no criming' rates remained high despite the policy changes and that further measures were required, together with a careful monitoring of police recording practices. The 1986 Home Office circular already referred to above (circular 69/86) recommended that complaints of rape and serious sexual assault should not be 'no crimed' unless there was a retraction of the complaint and an admission of fabrication by the complainant. This policy has subsequently been reinforced in a series of force orders. For example, in the Metropolitan Police Force (the Met.) serious offences against adults can only be 'no crimed' if 'there are substantial indications that the allegation is actually false' (Force Order CR 209/90/104(T)12). Our own research project, discussed in detail in subsequent chapters, was able to measure the impact of some of these more recent developments.

## Policing domestic violence

As domestic and sexual violence often occur together, it is impossible to provide a full assessment of police practices in relation to sexual assault without also considering the police response to domestic violence. If the rates of 'no criming' suggested that the police were not taking reports of rape and sexual assault seriously, then the extremely high rates of 'no criming' uncovered by Susan Edwards in her study of domestic violence gave even greater cause for concern, as they indicated that violence occurring in the private sphere between members of the same family or household was treated even more casually. Her research, undertaken in two police stations within the Metropolitan Police area (Hounslow and Holloway) and covering a six-month period during 1984 to 1985, found that out of 773 reported cases of domestic violence, a crime report was made in only 93, an incident report in a further 73 and several more were written up in the occurrence book. The use of this last category usually meant that further action was avoided. Of the 93 cases, 83 per cent were subsequently 'no crimed'; two-thirds of the 73 'incidents' were recorded as common assault and the victim advised to prosecute privately (Edwards 1989, chapter 4).

The author of the study found that the police tended to divert cases away from criminalization by avoiding making arrests, by referring parties to other agencies and by limiting their own involvement to stopping any violence actually in progress when they arrived. Of all the calls from the public in the domestic cases included in the study, 70 per cent were recorded as requiring 'no call for police action' and this formula was applied across a range of cases, including particularly difficult disputes. In 1986, the Met. produced their own report on domestic violence (Metropolitan Police 1986a) which, while not addressing the 'no criming' issue directly, did make a number of recommendations concerning the way that domestic violence was recorded and handled. In 1987 new guidelines were produced, giving a clear definition of domestic violence and this was followed by a force order emphasizing the need to improve training and reporting proce-dures, arrests and support to victims, stating unequivocally that 'an assault which occurs in the home is as much a criminal act as one which occurs in the street' (Edwards 1989: 199–200).

The domestic violence literature generally has documented how domestic cases are treated as 'rubbish' work by the police, who avoid arresting assaultive partners (McConville *et al.* 1991). Tony Faragher (1985) carried out one of the first observational studies. He obtained permission from the Staffordshire Police Force to observe their work and was on the scene of twenty-six domestic disputes. Not all the cases involved actual assault, but ten contained an infringement of the legal code, which could have formed the basis for a charge. Five of these involved assault, two were breaches of injunctions and the remaining three involved damage and/or theft by ex-husbands or ex-boyfriends. Of those cases where threats had been made against the woman's life, only 20 per cent saw an arrest made, and in cases where there was severe bruising the arrest rate was 15 per cent. Faragher concluded that the police were ineffective in enforcing injunctions and in assisting women householders to enforce them.

The police assumed that women would fail to co-operate in legal proceedings and would inevitably withdraw charges. However, this belief was not matched by the frequency with which this occurred in practice. Faragher concluded that 'the only way in which this low level of withdrawal can be accounted for is that the police were extremely selective about who they sponsor to take legal action'. This was confirmed by observation at the scene of 'domestics' where women were often asked if they really wanted to take action and were given time to 'think it over' in the belief that an 'unemotional' decision made later would be more realistic (Faragher 1985: 117).

In effect, the findings revealed that the police did not believe they should be concerned with the 'private domain' which had no public order implications. Reiner too found that domestic disputes, along with traffic control, were seen as frustrating 'because of their apparent uselessness from the standpoint of a specific notion of real police work' (Reiner 1978: 178). Faragher found that the focus was on maintaining public order rather than on the needs of the women complainants. He concluded that there was an urgent need for the area of work to be given higher status and for the introduction of training.

Police policy initiatives on domestic violence have only been in place nationally since 1990 in the UK (see Cromack 1995: 188) despite the numerous studies drawing attention to the shortcomings of police practice in this area. In 1990 an inter-agency working party was established to investigate domestic violence; in 1992 it produced a report containing recommendations on the co-ordination and extension of existing services. In August 1990 the Home Secretary announced that a higher priority would in future be given to domestic violence and that it would no longer be dismissed as not worthy of police time (Wolmar 1990). National guidelines were issued by the Home Office (circular 60/1990) recommending that all police officers should 'regard as their over-riding priority the protection of the victim and the apprehension of the offender'. The circular urged police forces to keep accurate records, enforce the criminal law and offer sympathetic treatment and support to victims. In the wake of these guidelines, specialized domestic violence units were established in some areas, enabling non-uniformed officers to follow up cases and co-ordinate services.

There is conflicting evidence with regard to how much police record keeping and general response to domestic violence has improved overall. Home Office research (Grace 1995) found that while nearly all police forces had formulated policies on domestic violence, emphasizing the importance of arresting the perpetrator, women's experiences of uniformed police were very mixed and in practice assailants were rarely arrested; for example the arrest rates were 13 per cent in Manchester, 18 per cent in Northumbria and 24 per cent in West Yorkshire. Over the past ten years, various home secretaries, the police, the CPS and the courts have all insisted that violent domestic assaults should be treated as seriously as crimes against strangers in the street. In practice, women subjected to violence are still given little protection and courts persist in treating offenders leniently. The myth that domestic assaults are not as serious as assaults by strangers is contested by the latest British Crime Survey (1996) which shows that on average domestic assaults have more serious consequences than non-domestic ones. A total of 69 per cent of domestic assaults result in injuries compared with 41 per cent for assaults on strangers; 'trivial' domestic attacks are very rarely reported.

In some areas, there is evidence of improvements in police practice, and Domestic Violence Units (DVUs) staffed by non-uniformed police officers provide some essential support for victims. Research suggests that police practice has improved in some areas but not in others. Hanmer and Saunders (1990) reported greater satisfaction with police treatment after the introduction of DVUs in West Yorkshire and Morley and Mullender (1994) found that women generally preferred dealing with the non-uniformed DVU officers. In her Islington study (1993), Jayne Mooney found that women who had sought help from the police since the implementation of the new policies were more satisfied with the treatment they received than were women who had been to the police prior to the policy changes. They reported that the police officers running the DVUs were supportive and helpful, but some women had difficulties getting in touch with the officers as telephone lines were constantly engaged; when police were called to an incident, response times were too slow and, apart from referring the woman to the DVU, the police still took little action at the scene. As Kelly *et al.* (1998) point out, it is not the role of DVUs to respond to domestic violence calls; in some cases officers do investigative work and help to develop local policies and practices, but mostly they provide various forms of support for complainants and keep records of assaults that have been reported. On the issue of record keeping, Grace (1995) found that many forces had problems compiling accurate records due no doubt to insufficient funding.

Little research has been conducted into the experience of black and ethnic minority women. Amina Mama's study (1989) is an exception. She undertook a study of women who had experienced violence in the home and highlighted three major areas of concern. First, she drew attention to the reluctance of black women to call in the police, even when serious and even life-threatening crimes were being committed. (However, this is contradicted by more recent studies which suggest that some black women are more likely to contact the police than white women as we shall see in Chapter 4.) Second, she identified a reluctance on the part of the police to enforce the law when they were called in. Third, she found examples of the police adding insult to injury by themselves behaving in an abusive manner towards the women. Despite the extreme violence suffered by most of the women interviewed, only a few had called the police on their own account. In many cases the call was made by someone else on their behalf.

The researchers point to the divided loyalties experienced by black women, particularly if they are in relationships with men whom they know to have experienced police harassment in the past. They refer to cases in which being called to the scene of domestic violence was used by the police as an excuse for assaulting a black man and cases in which the whole affair turned into an immigration investigation. A solicitor interviewed during the course of the research revealed that in some of her cases the police arrested the woman, pending inquiries into her immigration status (Mama 1989: 177). The researchers conclude that police responses were very mixed, ranging from being helpful and supportive, for example making contact with black women's centres or refuges, to placing the woman in even greater danger by being unsympathetic or even abusive.[2] The researchers emphasized the need for police training to include an understanding of racism and the need for better legal advice and support for black women to enable them to escape from violent situations.

An evaluation of domestic violence units by Cromack (1995), based on research in Hull, found little evidence of improvement in police practice since new policies had been introduced. She looked in particular at the police response to a pro-active arrest policy and concluded that the Home Office circular had as yet had little effect. Officers thought that it was a waste of time to prepare documentation if the victim was uncertain as to whether or not to proceed; arrest of offenders was generally avoided; officers found it hard to comprehend why women stayed in violent relationships and there was little awareness of how to monitor and follow up repeat victimization. Cromack's overall conclusion was that the problem was 'an underlying police culture that tends towards the belief that domestic violence is a private family matter and more appropriately a subject for civil law' (1995: 197). Research undertaken on behalf of the *Dispatches* television programme (1998) found that many domestic violence units were only employing one officer and were run on a shoe string; some police divisions had not established units at all.

In their evaluation report on the Domestic Violence Matters project carried out in two London boroughs, Liz Kelly *et al.* (1998) found that in the six months immediately prior to the setting up of the project in 1993 almost two-thirds of domestic violence incidents were not recorded as crimes and of the total arrests, charges were laid in less than half (47 per cent). This was just over one-sixth of the offences which were crimed. During the period covered by the pilot study, a higher proportion of cases were recorded as crimes but the findings on the rate of arrests were inconclusive.

## Domestic violence in the courts

The Crown Prosecution Service discontinues cases more often in domestic than non-domestic cases. The Home Affairs Select Committee 1993 explained this in the following terms:

> The CPS is not immune to the difficulties of balancing one aspect of the public interest, which rightly condemns personal violence in any form, with another strand of public interest which recognizes the benefit of preserving the family unit, wherever possible.

This policy has serious consequences. Cretney and Davis (1996, 1997) carried out an extensive study of the police and CPS handling of domestic violence cases in Avon and Somerset focusing particularly on the way the police, CPS and courts 'manage' the reluctant victim and on the compellability provision whereby a wife can now be compelled to give evidence against her husband (see Police and Criminal Evidence Act 1984, Section 80). They found no improvement in the prosecution process. Defence lawyers who sought to have the charges dropped were likely to paint a picture of restored domestic harmony, or alternatively, they might suggest that the accusation is made by a woman scorned or by a jealous or alcoholic woman. A variety of tactics were employed by defence barristers to divert attention from the violence. Mild language was used when referring to the degree of disharmony between the woman and her assailant and strong language when referring to the character of the complainant. Cretney and Davis point to the shortcomings of the adversarial process, whereby only the bare outline of the incident is presented in court even though it represents the culmination of years of violence. They analyzed why sentences were so low for offences involving such serious levels of violence and concluded that what crucially determined sentence length was not the gravity of the offence, but whether or not the defendant was still seen as part of 'the couple'. Where the relationship had ended, offenders were much more likely to go to prison; where it was said that the two were still a 'couple', the offender would receive a fine or a conditional discharge. Some magistrates defended lenient sentences on the grounds that they did not want to punish the victim as well as the offender. However, such practices acted as an incentive for the defence to present the court with a misleading picture of domestic harmony and resulted in high levels of dissatisfaction among complainants. Many of the women interviewed had hoped that their assailant would receive some kind of treatment to help him control his violent behaviour. Most assault victims concluded that the court was not a place where their problems could be satisfactorily addressed.

## Legislative developments

### Police powers and law relating to domestic violence

During the 1980s, police powers were increased, particularly in relation to public order offences. The Police and Criminal Evidence Act (PACE) 1984 provides for the 'stop and search' of persons or vehicles if the officer has 'reasonable grounds' for suspecting that a crime has been committed (section 1). An officer may also enter premises without a warrant for the purposes of 'saving life or limb' (section 17) and can make an arrest where necessary 'to protect a child or other vulnerable person from the relevant person' (section 25). As Susan Edwards (1989) argued, potentially these powers could be used to protect women subjected to violence. Section 80 of PACE empowered the courts to compel a husband or wife to give evidence against the other spouse. If used insensitively, however, it could place women in even greater danger from violent husbands while also incurring the wrath of the court if the women refused to give evidence. However, research by Cretney and Davis (1996) found that the compellability provision was almost never used. Very occasionally the non-married have been compelled to give evidence as epitomized by the case of Michelle Renshaw, committed to prison for refusing to give evidence against the boyfriend charged with attacking her. Edwards also argues that the cumulative effect of PACE, public order, picketing and industrial relations legislation in recent years has been to prioritize crimes occurring in the public as opposed to the private sphere, to focus attention on civil disorder and street crime and away from less visible acts such as male violence against women.

The Family Law Act 1996 was intended to give greater protection to victims of domestic violence. It streamlined the processes for applying for civil injunctions and was aimed at ensuring that police powers of arrest are attached to the majority of such injunctions. In future, if injunctions are breached, abusers will increasingly face the sanctions of the criminal law.[3] The Act also made provision for protection orders to be available from a single court for both married women and cohabitees. It amended the Children Act 1989 by making it possible to exclude an abuser from the home through interim care orders or emergency protection orders. These orders are to be made if the court is reasonably satisfied that the exclusion would prevent the child from suffering significant harm while enabling the caring parent to remain in the home and provide reasonable care (Radford 1996).

A particular area of concern is the trend for the courts to order contact to be made between violent fathers and their children after divorce or separation. The Children Act 1989, which came into effect in 1991, is based on the presumption that wherever possible children should retain contact with both parents. This reinforces the abuse of children and women through the legal presumption that parents should in almost all cases have contact with their children on divorce and separation, even when violence and abuse have occurred. In the case of violent fathers, this presumption has recently been challenged. A survey by the National Children's Home in 1997 highlighted the negative impact on children of violence perpetrated against their mothers. It concluded that steps towards greater intervention in relation to criminal law sanctions are being undermined by the Children Act because of its failure to acknowledge domestic violence. The supposed focus on the welfare of the child, defined in practice as contact with the absent male partner, operates to undermine the safety of women and children. Hester and Radford (1996) recommend a presumption of no contact in circumstances of domestic violence with the possibility of contact only if this can be arranged safely for both mother and child.

The situation for women faced with contact applications from violent fathers has become worse as they are now threatened with imprisonment if they refuse to comply (see Anderson 1997). In a case in January 1996, a woman from Newcastle was threatened with imprisonment for refusing to allow contact between her ex-husband and two children aged 9 and 7, although he had recently been released from prison following a six year sentence for raping and buggering her after a long history of violence towards her. In October 1996 Dawn Austin was imprisoned for contempt of court for obstructing contact between her ex-partner and two children. He had served a prison sentence for breaking her jaw and the court accepted when making the committal order that he had a history of serious violence (see *A v. N* (1997) 1 *Family Law Review* 533). Dawn Austin is a member of AMICA (Aid for Mothers Involved in Contact Cases), a network of women imprisoned or threatened with imprisonment for refusing contact in similar circumstances. It is significant that in the National Children's Home survey (1997) more than four out of five children were worried about domestic violence. The Rights of Women (ROW) pressure group set up a Best Interest Campaign with the aim of establishing the legal principle against violent and abusive parents having contact with their children on divorce or separation unless contact can be proven to be safe for any family member who might be affected.

## Child abuse and the law

There have been four major child abuse scandals in England and Wales in the 1980s and early 1990s in Leeds, Cleveland, the Orkneys and Wales. The first occurred in Leeds where seventeen sex rings were uncovered, involving twenty-one men who were ultimately prosecuted. More than two thousand children aged between 8 and 16 were involved. According to Campbell (1997), 'it was one of the biggest rings ever discovered in Britain and consumed the working, waking and sometimes sleeping lives of the police team involving five members for two years' (ibid. 105). It led to the creation of three specialist child protection units. In Cleveland, the media image of 121 children being snatched from their homes led to the Butler Schloss enquiry, which concluded that there was no reason to doubt the medical diagnosis (Campbell 1997). In 1992 the National Society for the Prevention of Cruelty to Children published a report on *Child Sexual Abuse Trends in England and Wales* which investigated 10,000 children on their 'at risk' register. In the same year Lord Clyde's report of the inquiry into the Orkneys condemned the removal of children from their homes in dawn raids following suspicion of satanic abuse and called for procedures and guidelines on sexual abuse to be developed.

The most shocking report of a child abuse scandal in Britain occurred in 1997, when a tribunal of inquiry into child abuse in Chester heard 300 adult survivors of alleged sexual abuse bear witness against 148 adults, mainly professional child care staff who had sexually assaulted them as children. The Utting report (1997) presents a picture of runaway children often returned to their abusers; many were not believed and were subjected to bullying and intimidation. The police played a central role and indeed initiated the investigation in Wales.

Growing public awareness of the threat that paedophiles pose to children in view of the very high rates of recidivism has become an issue both in Britain and the United States. Police stations in the US publicly display lists of convicted paedophiles and when an offender is released the police have an obligation to inform neighbours. In Britain the police can now use their discretion as to whether or not neighbours should be informed. The Sexual Offenders Act 1997 creates a national register of people convicted of sexual crimes and makes it compulsory for all offenders with convictions for sexual offences to register with the police so that their whereabouts are known.

## Law reform in relation to rape and sexual assault

The judicial treatment of rape has undergone some changes in the past twenty years, mainly in response to the campaigning of groups such as the Rights of Women, the Women's Aid Federation, Women Against Rape and Rape Crisis groups; also in the light of growing evidence of the inadequacy of the present judicial system, as highlighted for example by Detective Inspector Blair (1985).[4] As long ago as 1975, the Advisory Group on the Law of Rape (the Heilbron Committee) concluded that the way in which defence lawyers challenged the credibility of complainants by delving into their past sexual history was unacceptable; it did nothing to advance the cause of justice while effectively putting the woman on trial. Accordingly, the Sexual Offences (Amendment) Act 1976 was passed with the intention of limiting the use of such evidence. Under section 2, the defence is required to apply to the judge for permission to cross-examine the complainant regarding her sexual history or sexual character. It was left to the discretion of the judge to decide this issue, so that in practice, this section appears to have had little effect (see Adler 1987, Temkin 1993). Also under this Act, complainants were for the first time provided with anonymity in media coverage of rape cases, from the moment that someone was charged with the offence. The same anonymity was also given to the accused, although the Heilbron Committee had not considered this necessary; in 1988 this symmetry was broken when the protection for complainants was increased and that for defendants was removed (see below).

Other changes to rape legislation in Britain in recent years have in general taken the form of widening both the definition of rape and the circumstances in which it is recognized to have occurred. In England and Wales, the common law presumption that a boy under 14 years of age is incapable of sexual intercourse was abolished as a result of a private member's bill in 1993. In Scotland, the marital rape exemption was gradually removed through case law, culminating in a judgment that a man could be charged with raping his wife when they were still living together (*Stallard* v. *HM Advocate* 1989 SCCR 248). English law followed suit two years later in the case of *R* v. *R*, in which the House of Lords held that 'in modern times the supposed marital exemption in rape forms no part of the law of England' (*R* v. *R* [1991] 3 WLR 767). This change in case law was enshrined in statute in the Criminal Justice and Public Order Act 1994. The implication of the marital rape exclusion was that a husband had the right to sexual intercourse whenever he chose, a reflection of the historical domination of husbands over wives. Its abolition carries the clear implication that wives have a right to self determination. At the same time, the definition of rape was widened to include non-consensual buggery of men. This was the first time rape of men was acknowledged. In June 1995 a historical breakthrough occurred with the first conviction for male rape under the new law.

In response to public outrage at lenient sentences imposed by a number of judges in rape cases, a private member's bill in 1985 increased the maximum penalty for attempted rape from seven years to life, so that attempted rape as well as actual rape could in theory attract a life sentence (Sexual Offences Act 1985 section 3). The same piece of legislation also raised the maximum penalty for indecent assault on women from two years to ten years, thereby bringing it into line with the penalty for indecent assault on boys and men (section 3). This recognition of the serious nature of these crimes was reinforced the following year when the Lord Chief Justice issued new sentencing guidelines for judges dealing with cases of rape. This move followed in the wake of a number of well-publicized cases of extreme judicial leniency towards rapists which had provoked a public outcry, together with the revelation in the 1984 criminal statistics that only 8 per cent of convicted rapists were imprisoned for more than five years. Giving judgment in the case of Billam ([1986] 1 All ER 985), Lord Chief Justice Lane indicated that there should be a minimum sentence of five years for adult rapists pleading not guilty in cases with no mitigating circumstances. Eight years should be the minimum where two or more rapists acted together, for men who burgled as well as raped, for men who abused positions of responsibility and for those who abducted their victims.

A number of changes in the law have given more prominence to the victims of crime (see Mawby and Walklate 1994). The Criminal Justice Act 1982 made it clear that in cases where the court had ordered compensation for the victim but also imposed a fine, compensation was to take priority. The Criminal Justice Act 1988 required courts to give reasons why they had not ordered compensation to be paid in circumstances where they could have done this. It also removed the right of the accused to anonymity, while extending anonymity for the complainant from the moment of reporting. Such legislative changes were supplemented by the publication of the Victim's Charter by the Home Office in 1990, which included recommendations designed to improve the treatment of victims by the judicial system.

Another major obstacle to securing a conviction in rape and sexual assault trials has been the existence of the corroboration rule, which required the judge in a sexual offence trial to warn the jury of the danger of convicting on the evidence of the complainant alone. Since the passing of the Criminal Justice and Public Order Act 1994, it is no longer mandatory for judges to give the corroboration warning but is left to their discretion. Unfortunately it is unlikely to be any more effective that the Sexual Offences (Amendment) Act 1976, which was designed to limit the introduction of sexual history evidence, but which judges have continued to allow (see Adler 1993, Lees 1997a). According to Helen Grindrod QC (interview, September 1997) the corroboration warning is still invariably given in Britain despite direction from the Court of Appeal that it should only be given in exceptional circumstances (for discussion of this see Lees 1997a: 251). In Canada and New South Wales the corroboration requirement has been abolished altogether. In any event, it seems likely that the police and the CPS will continue to ensure that cases in which there is no corroborative evidence, traditionally regarded as 'weak' cases, are dropped long before they reach the stage of a jury trial.

The Criminal Justice and Public Order Act 1994 also modified the defendant's right to silence. Where defendants refuse to testify, judges now have discretion to direct the jury to draw inferences from this silence. These changes are unlikely to have any effect on shifting the current imbalance in rape and sexual assault trials so heavily weighted in favour of the accused. As we shall see, in recent years it appears to have become even more difficult to gain convictions in such trials. Jennifer Temkin (1993) showed how appeal court decisions had led to problems in implementing the Sexual Offences Amendment Act 1976. Sue Lees (1997a) monitored all the trials of rape and attempted rape at two Crown Courts over a four month period in 1994 and found that serial rapists were regularly acquitted. She proposed a package of reforms to reverse the imbalances in trials and called for the monitoring of trials, and greater accountability and training for all criminal justice professionals.

### The law on sexual harassment

Since the mid-1980s, feminist lawyers have been able to persuade industrial tribunals that sexual harassment is a form of sex discrimination prohibited by the Sex Discrimination Act 1975 (Gregory 1995). This has been reinforced by developments in European law, notably the Recommendation and Code of Practice on sexual harassment (European Commission 1992) and the abolition of the ceiling on compensation awards in discrimination cases (see Chapter 2 note 2), which has resulted in a steady rise in levels of compensation awarded to successful complainants in sexual harassment cases.

The Criminal Justice and Public Order Act 1994 made intentional harassment in the street and at work a criminal offence for the first time, including harassment on the grounds of race, sex, sexuality and disability (section 154). A private member's bill to deal with stalking became the Protection from Harassment Act 1997, making harassment a criminal offence and a civil tort, enabling anyone who suffers alarm or distress from such harassment to obtain an injunction and damages against the harasser. This legislation was precipitated by the case of Dennis Chambers who, defending himself, was allowed to sit at the front of the court rather than in the dock, which brought him closer to the woman whom he had allegedly stalked for four years (*The Times*, 25 September 1996).

Despite the continuing emphasis on violence in the public sphere, these developments do increase the legal ammunition available to women suffering various forms of sexual violence. By invoking criminal sanctions, these laws will require the active involvement and commitment of the police to be fully effective. So far, the police seem to have responded more enthusiastically to the concept of 'zero tolerance' as propounded by the New York police, involving the zealous policing of petty vandals and graffiti artists, rather than giving their support to the feminist 'zero tolerance' campaign. This latter was a poster campaign launched in major cities throughout Britain from 1993 onwards, co-ordinated by the National Association of Local Government Women's Committees and supported by feminist activist groups. The theme of the campaign was the unacceptability of domestic violence, with slogans such as: 'he gave her chocolates, flowers and multiple bruising' and 'behind these great men are the women they battered' (*Rights of Women Bulletin*, Spring 1994).

## Policing sexual assault

The police exercise a considerable degree of discretion in the course of their work, including when making decisions in relation to cases of rape and sexual assault. In recent years, they have been made increasingly aware of the importance of service delivery to complainants, but they also have to deal with the Crown Prosecution Service, which has its own agenda and which is in turn heavily influenced by what is happening in the courts. Effecting radical change in police policies and practices in relation to crimes of violence is therefore only one stage in the process of securing justice for those on the receiving end of this violence. It is, however, a crucial first step, precisely because the police do represent the status quo. The challenge for feminists is to take advantage of the current emphasis on law and order in order to highlight the endemic nature of male violence, without endorsing the more reactionary implications of policies rooted in notions of social control and social exclusion. The police are not the most obvious allies to assist in this endeavour. As we demonstrate in Chapter 2, the prevalence of a macho culture within the police force has allowed male violence to thrive within its ranks and created resistance to equal opportunities policies imposed from above. Unless rapid progress is made towards putting their own house in order, policy changes currently being implemented by the police in relation to male violence will be little more than cosmetic.

The remaining chapters draw on our own research in order to evaluate recent changes in the policing of rape and sexual assault. Chapter 3 focuses on police practices in relation to recording and classifying reports of sexual attacks. It also explores the implications of the separation between the roles of investigation and prosecution with the creation of the Crown Prosecution Service and provides a critical examination of the work of the Service, drawing on our own findings and on the experiences of feminist practitioners working in this area. Chapter 4 continues the exploration of the reasons for the high rates of attrition in cases of rape and sexual assault, seeking to identify which cases are most likely to fall away and at which points in the criminal justice process this attrition occurs. Comparing our own findings with those of the Home Office study by Grace *et al.* (1992), we assess the impact of any prior relationship between the suspects and complainants (and of particular characteristics of both) on case outcomes. We attempt to unravel the evidence on the ethnicity of complainants and suspects and the relevance of this information for the way that reported cases of rape are processed.

Following the widening of the definition of rape in the Criminal Justice and Public Order Act 1994 to include non-consensual penetration of the anus, Chapter 5 reports on the first survey of police recording practices of assaults by men on men. This research, undertaken for a Channel 4 *Dispatches* programme 'Male Rape' makes it possible to begin to analyze some of the characteristics of assailants and victims, such as sexual orientation, and their relationship to each other. Analysis of this relationship is, however, limited by inadequate police recording practices. Continuing with the theme of service delivery, Chapters 6 and 7 report on the experiences of women complainants, their views of the police response to their complaint and of the medical examination and, for those whose cases went to court, their experiences of that process. We also examine the role of other agencies such as Rape Crisis and Victim Support and other counselling and medical services. The final chapter assesses the achievements and shortcomings of the last two decades with regard to policing practices and the operation of the criminal justice system. It re-examines the laws relating to rape and sexual assault and their implementation, drawing on the experiences of other countries in order to focus attention on the need for radical reform in this country.

# 2   Police culture and its contradictions

## Introduction

In her book *No Way up the Greasy Pole*, Alison Halford describes her career in the police force and in particular the events surrounding her complaint of sex discrimination against the police and the Home Office after nine separate applications for promotion had proved unsuccessful. She begins with an account of a bizarre procedure which she encountered when she applied to enter the Metropolitan Police in the early 1960s at the age of 22:

> The women [candidates] were lined up alongside each other and paraded in front of a mixed panel of very senior police officers who instructed us to remove all our upper clothing – bras as well. Then we were given a looking over and expected, in this highly vulnerable state of undress, to answer a series of questions put by a po-faced panel of experienced police officers.
>
> (Halford 1993: 17)

She admits that no female recruit would have to undergo such an undignified ordeal nowadays, but in view of the failure of police women to break through the glass ceiling into the higher echelons of the police force in any significant numbers and also in view of the growing number of reports of sexual harassment and even of rape of women officers by their male colleagues, it is important to consider just how far reaching these procedural changes have been.

The changes that have occurred are a direct result of the passing of the Equal Pay Act 1970 and the Sex Discrimination Act 1975 (both of which came into force in 1975), making it illegal for employers to discriminate against women in their terms and conditions of employment and requiring them to provide equal opportunities in regard to recruitment, access to promotion and other benefits. Exemptions for the police service were limited to requirements relating to height, uniform and equipment and special treatment for women in connection with pregnancy and childbirth. As Sandra Jones points out, these exemptions were intended to protect women against discrimination by recognizing biological differences, including the fact that the average woman is shorter than the average man (Jones 1986). Senior police officers and the Police Federation were united in their opposition to the legislation and lobbied hard for an exemption along similar lines to the exemption granted to the Armed Forces, but this was denied.[1]

The 1970s sex discrimination legislation was designed to tackle job segregation across the labour market and particularly to open up male-dominated areas of work to women. Similarly, the Race Relations Act 1976 addressed the issue of race discrimination at work. The laws also extended beyond employment and sought to ensure equal treatment for women and for minority racial and ethnic groups in the provision of goods, facilities and services. They were therefore just as important in raising questions about the ways in which the police delivered services to the public as in requiring a re-examination of employment practices. The relationship between these two aspects of the legislation may not have been immediately apparent in the 1970s, but since then there has been a growing recognition that a police force which consists almost entirely of white males will lack credibility in its dealings with those outside this elite group (Smith and Gray 1985, Dunhill 1989, Hanmer *et al.* 1989, Holdaway 1996). Nevertheless, at the most senior level, police officers have proven extremely resistant to the introduction of measures which would help to achieve radical change within the service, so that progress towards equal opportunities is painfully slow; it is largely driven by litigation from the ranks rather than by positive initiatives from senior officers.

## Equality or difference?

The initial and continuing resistance to allowing women to be employed within the police force on the same terms as men is deeply rooted in the structure and culture of the force. During the nineteenth century, only 'fit men' could become police officers and the early policewomen were volunteers, emerging during the First World War specifically to protect the moral well-being of girls and young women, particularly from licentious soldiers (Jones 1986: 2). After the war, the first paid women officers were employed by the Metropolitan Police, with Home Office approval, in special Women Police Patrols. Small

numbers of policewomen continued to be employed at the discretion
of local police authorities, mainly in separate departments and mainly
for duties concerning women and children. During the Second World
War their numbers and range of duties increased, but by 1971 they still
constituted less than four per cent of the total person power and the
sexual division of labour persisted, so that they were largely confined
to duties involving female offenders, child neglect and other family
matters (Jones 1986: 5).

In order to comply with the equal opportunities legislation, during
the early part of the 1970s policewomen were awarded equal pay with
male officers; their separate departments were disbanded and they
were formally integrated into the mainstream of police duties. If
policewomen gave these changes a rather lukewarm welcome, it was
partly because the move to equality required them to adapt totally to
male patterns of working, including shift work. There was a recognition that promotion chances would be reduced with the abolition of
the specialist women's departments, as the women were only too aware
that they would meet discrimination when competing for 'male' jobs.
There was also a genuine concern that expertise in relation to their
service role would become dissipated. The majority of policemen were
even more appalled, as women in the force had only been tolerated
while the majority of them were confined to their separate ghetto of
departments and duties. In the words of the Police Federation representative: 'the very nature of the duties of a police constable is
contrary to all that is finest and best in women.' (Whittaker 1979,
quoted in Jones 1986: 8).

The belief that policework is essentially masculine and that women
are therefore unsuited to it, apart from a few low status areas of work
where their 'natural' caring and listening skills may be usefully
harnessed, is still the prevalent view within the police force today. It
explains why women still only constitute some 14 per cent of the force
and are concentrated in the lower grades and in certain specialist areas
of work. Sandra Jones uncovered an informal 10 per cent quota of
female recruits operating in the Midlands force where she undertook
her research in the early 1980s (Jones 1986) and Smith and Gray (1985)
reported the same finding in their study of the Metropolitan Police.
Smith and Gray found that the chances of acceptance into the force
were two and a half times higher for men than for women applicants;
they were told that 'operational considerations' made the unofficial
(and illegal) quota necessary. These considerations were based on the
assumption that women are unsuited to handling public order events
or incidents where violence is anticipated.

In 1980, Marguerite Johnston, who had been employed as a full time member of the Royal Ulster Constabulary (RUC) Reserve on a fixed-term contract, brought a sex discrimination case against the Chief Constable of the RUC for failure to renew her contract. His reason for non-renewal was that a substantial part of general police duties involved the use of fire-arms and his policy was not to issue women officers with firearms or train them in their use. He argued that if women officers were armed, it would increase the risk of their becoming targets for assassination; that armed female officers would be less effective in areas for which women are 'better suited', such as welfare work dealing with families and children; and that if women were to carry fire-arms it would be regarded by the public as a much greater departure from the ideal of an unarmed police force (see Equal Opportunities Review, July/August 1986, 8: 31).

Before the hearing, the Secretary of State for Northern Ireland issued a certificate under the exemption in the Sex Discrimination (N. Ireland) Order for actions done to safeguard national security and protect public safety and public order. Mrs Johnson's lawyers argued that no such exemption existed in European law. The case was referred to the European Court of Justice (ECJ), which found in her favour ([1986] Industrial Relations Law Reports (IRLR) 263 ECJ). Although the European Equal Treatment Directive allows exemptions for the protection of women, these are narrowly interpreted to refer to biological differences such as pregnancy and maternity and the Court has not allowed them to provide an excuse for excluding women from forms of employment merely because they may be considered 'unfeminine'. This decision made it clear that women could not be excluded from the police force, nor from certain areas of work within it, on the grounds that they needed to be protected. It was, however, very much a case of equality for women on men's terms; those women who could emulate male working patterns had the best chance of surviving as police officers. Nothing in the ECJ decision required the police to re-examine their employment practices, nor to abandon their stereotypical ideas of appropriate male and female behaviour. Also, seven years elapsed before the RUC took steps to arm women officers.

A number of studies of the police have commented on the strong male culture that exists within the force. Despite the fact that a substantial minority of police officers are women, Smith and Gray found that the dominant values were still those of an all-male institution such as a rugby club or boys' school. This manifests itself in a variety of ways:

in the emphasis on remaining dominant in any encounter and not losing face, the emphasis placed on masculine solidarity and on backing up other men in the group, especially when they are in the wrong, the stress on drinking as a test of manliness and a basis for good fellowship, the importance given to physical courage and the glamour attached to violence. This set of attitudes and norms amounts to a 'cult of masculinity', which also has a strong influence on policemen's behaviour towards women, towards victims of sexual offences and towards sexual offenders.

(Smith and Gray 1985: 372)

While such a culture persists, women officers are confronted by an impossible dilemma; they either become defeminized or deprofessionalized. If they perform their work competently, they are no longer seen as women; if they adopt subordinate roles and collude with male definitions of male and female roles, they cannot fulfil their potential as police officers (Bryant *et al.* 1985). A similar study of police officers serving in the RUC concluded that policewomen either became 'one of the boys' or they became victims, 'suffering in silence'. Those who accepted the feminine role as defined for them by the occupational culture merely succeeded in attracting even more sexual horseplay from the men (Brewer 1991). In the course of her interviews with policemen, Sandra Jones was provided with a number of anecdotes about individual policewomen who were perfectly capable of coping with public order situations. Although the women's skills were grudgingly acknowledged by the men, they responded by giving them derogatory nicknames and by continuing to question the morality of exposing women to high risk situations. The men also insisted that in a violent situation, a woman colleague could put a male officer at risk, either through not being able to provide backup or because he felt bound, out of chivalry, to protect her and so put himself at risk.

The contrary viewpoint was expressed forcefully by one of the women police constables (WPCs) taking part in the research conducted by Bryant *et al.*:

It has been found that WPCs can use charm and common sense to such a degree that the need for physical strength never arises and that some male officers often provoke volatile situations that should never occur.

(Bryant *et al.* 1985: 241)

The notion that women are necessarily better than men at defusing violent situations merely involves exchanging one set of stereotypes for another, whereas the real issue is to identify the best selection procedures and the appropriate training mechanisms to ensure that all police officers, regardless of sex, are able to handle public order situations satisfactorily.

The irony of the controversy concerning the suitability of women for police work is that it has taken place against the background of a major transformation in the common sense understanding of the police officer's role. Although most front-line policemen continue to characterize their work as tough, physical and dangerous, this perception is increasingly at odds with the public recognition of the police as providers of a wide range of services. A dramatic shift has occurred, from the concept of a police 'force' to that of a police 'service' (Reiner 1992). Robert Reiner writes of the gradual acceptance of this shift at senior levels and its continued resistance by the operational ranks, who complain that the emphasis on community policing detracts from the real police work of fighting crime (ibid. 141). Reiner's contribution to the debate is to argue that most police work is neither social service nor law enforcement, but order maintenance: the settlement of conflicts by means other than formal law enforcement. He writes: 'The craft of effective policing is to use the background possibility of legitimate coercion so skilfully that it never needs to be foregrounded', although he adds that the handling of domestic disputes as noncriminal, order-maintenance matters has been criticized by feminists and led to a shift back towards law enforcement for this category of calls (ibid. 143).

If Reiner's analysis is correct, it would suggest that women have a major role to play in the modern day police force. With appropriate training, there is no area of work that they are not competent to handle; in addition, they have an important role to play in relation to crimes against women and children, where the complainants need to reveal intimate and distressing details and often express a preference for a female officer.

## The limited impact of equal opportunities policies

Despite the lip service paid to equal opportunities in the higher echelons of the police force, the overall response continues to be patchy. A steady stream of evidence points to the persistence of employment practices and cultural attitudes which prevent women from making progress within the force. Bryant *et al.* (1985) investigated the reasons for the high turnover rate of women officers and found that many became disillusioned because of the numerous obstacles to career progression they encountered. One officer reported being asked at her promotion board when she intended to give up work and start a family. Not only is this line of questioning illegal under the Sex Discrimination Act, it reflects the persistence of deeply entrenched and outdated attitudes towards working women and of inflexible working practices which take no account of the possibilities of career breaks, job sharing or part time working. Without such schemes, the wastage of talent will continue unabated, as women are forced to choose between family and career, a choice that men are not required to make.

More recently, Carol Martin's investigation into the implementation of equal opportunities policies in one division of the Sussex Police found that women officers showed no desire to climb the promotional ladder. Several of them had applied to join the Special Inquiry Unit, dealing with sexual and child abuse. This enabled them to work along-side other women officers, and at the same time escape from a hostile working environment elsewhere, but it simultaneously reduced their chances of promotion, as the work was regarded as low status, despite its investigative nature, no doubt because of the predominance of female officers within it. One WPC commented:

> When I first joined I was very promotion-minded. I was going to be a superintendent, but after a long time in the job I realise that I'm just not a leader of people. I just wouldn't want the extra burden of other people – I've got enough on my own plate to be honest.
>
> (Martin 1996: 517)

Martin suggests that this deflating of the women's ambitions is culturally produced by their experiences within the force. For example, during training they are often reprimanded for being too aggressive, although male trainees will be rewarded for the same behaviour, which is then redefined as assertiveness. Martin concludes:

> Women who joined with a positive and assertive view soon realised that this could cause them difficulties, and adapted to fit in with the cultural expectations which existed for WPCs.
>
> (Martin 1996: 518)

This interpretation is supported by the findings of an earlier study undertaken in the United States, which found that the longer women remained in the force, the more likely they were to revise their career expectations in a downwards direction (Poole and Pogrebin 1988). It seems that they were deterred both by the absence of female role models – an indication of the difficulties of securing promotion – and by the prospect of having to prove themselves all over again in a supervisory role, after working long and hard to be accepted in the lower ranks.

On a practical level, Martin found no consideration on the part of the Sussex Police of how to resolve the work/family dilemma:

> Many of the [women] talked about wasting talented officers who cannot return to their jobs after maternity leave because of the existing structure. This issue was seen as the burning question, which has the greatest significance for most potential and existing female police officers, and one that has been completely sidestepped by existing equal opportunities policies.
>
> (Martin 1996: 521)

It is not that the police do not respond to criticisms, but rather that they do not enquire deeply enough into the underlying causes of the problems that have been identified, so that the proposed solutions do not go far enough. In the mid-1980s, the Metropolitan Police responded to the revelations of Smith and Gray (1985) concerning the existence of illegal recruitment quotas (see above). The revelations were made in a research study which Scotland Yard had itself commissioned from the Policy Studies Institute (PSI), arising chiefly from a concern about the quality of police relations with ethnic minority groups. Around the same time, Scotland Yard also agreed to undertake a joint exercise with the Equal Opportunities Commission (EOC).

The trigger for this second investigation was the tribunal case of *de Launay* v. *Commissioner of Police for the Metropolis*. In 1983, WPC de Launay had been banned from working with a married PC on traffic patrol duties following a rumour that they were having a sexual relationship. There was no real evidence that this was the case, but apparently the chief superintendent was concerned that, as they were 'both attractive people' (Jones 1986: 147), such a relationship was likely to develop. A new rule was introduced that female officers should not be given permanent patrols with married men. As there was only one unmarried male officer at the garage where Wendy de Launay worked, this effectively made it impossible for the three female officers based there to continue with their duties. After filing her complaint of unlawful sex discrimination, WPC de Launay was moved to foot patrol

duties. The tribunal made a finding of sex discrimination and victimization, but went on to reprimand both the chief superintendent and
the complainant for not taking appropriate steps to resolve the matter
internally. It was left to the parties to the dispute to consider what
action needed to be taken (Tina Martin 1996). The collaborative investigation with the EOC formed part of the subsequent agreement.

In the report which resulted, the PSI finding of an unofficial quota,
restricting the recruitment of women to 10 per cent, was confirmed. The
investigators also found that women were excluded from certain areas,
such as the mounted police and diplomatic protection and were unlikely
to be deployed on public order duties (EOC/Metropolitan Police 1989).
As a result of the findings, a big recruitment drive increased the proportion of female recruits to 30 per cent, but no practical steps were taken
to ensure that those recruits entered a working environment in which
their skills and enthusiasm could be fully utilized. A study undertaken
in Scotland around the same time found similar patterns of discrimination within Scottish police forces (Centre for Police Studies 1989).

As a consequence of the PSI study and while the EOC investigation
was still underway, the Metropolitan Police formed an equal opportunities working party and by December 1986 a formal equal
opportunities policy had been produced. A comprehensive document
*Equal Opportunities Guidelines for Police Managers* was distributed to
all officers of the rank of inspector and above. This work provided the
basis for Home Office Circular 87/1989 issued to all police forces in
England and Wales in November 1989, so that by March 1992, all
forces had published equal opportunities policies and associated
grievance procedures (Tina Martin 1996).

Statements of intent enshrined in equal opportunities policies are
easy to make; implementing them in the face of widespread hostility
and resistance is a different matter. Alison Halford filed her sex
discrimination complaint in May 1990, some months after the Home
Office guidelines had been circulated. With the backing of the Equal
Opportunities Commission, she complained that Northamptonshire
Police Authority had failed to shortlist her for the post of Deputy
Chief Constable (DCC), although three less experienced men had been
shortlisted. Her superiors responded by subjecting her to disciplinary
proceedings and only after what Halford describes as two years of
vilification and humiliation in an attempt to make her drop the case,
culminating in two weeks' gruelling cross-examination in the tribunal,
did they agree to settle. In exchange for £15,000, she was to take early
retirement on 'medical grounds' with a full pension. The case, which
had seemed quite straightforward at the outset, had absorbed more

than half the EOC's annual legal budget and deprived Ms Halford of the career she loved, all because she had dared to try to climb the 'greasy pole' (Halford 1993).

As Lorraine Paddison explains, there were no winners in this scenario, only losers:

> The 39 days of evidence provided the press with many column inches of lurid insights into the lives of senior officers on Merseyside – 'liquidaceous' dinners attended by senior officers and the so-called 'canteen culture' of the force in which sexist and racist views and behaviour appear commonplace. As the costs escalated, as the image of the police plummeted and Halford became worn down with the pressure of the case, the parties finally settled.
>
> (Paddison 1992: 6)

This was not the end of the litigation arising from this case, however, as Alison Halford decided to complain to the European Court of Human Rights about the bugging of her office telephone by fellow officers, something she became aware of shortly after filing her discrimination complaint. She complained that the interception of her calls amounted to an unjustifiable interference with her rights to respect for her private life and freedom of expression (as required by Article 8 of the European Convention on Human Rights) and that she had no effective domestic remedy (as required by Article 13), because there was no provision in national law to regulate internal communications systems operated by public authorities, such as the Merseyside Police. In June 1997 the Court found in her favour, holding that the interception of Ms Halford's calls

> was a serious infringement of the applicant's rights, bearing in mind that it appeared to have been carried out by the police with the primary purpose of gathering material to be used against her in sex discrimination proceedings.
>
> ([1997] IRLR 471)

Ms Halford commented:

> When it comes to tapping phones in this country the law as it stands indicates that you must be a terrorist, a subversive or a threat to the public. Bringing an equality action did not put me in that category.
>
> (*Guardian*, 26 June 1997)

Alison Halford was not the only policewoman who had decided that enough was enough. In December 1989, a WPC had resigned from the Bedfordshire Police after four years, alleging that she was 'repeatedly called "an old dog" and hounded out of her job by a campaign of verbal sexual abuse'. Two years later, a female member of the Diplomatic Protection Squad took the Metropolitan Police to an industrial tribunal on the grounds that dress regulations forced her, unlike her male colleagues, to carry her gun in her handbag. The same officer was also instrumental in persuading the Met. to supply female firearm officers with body armour which was tailored for women (*Guardian*, 6 February 1993).

As part of the settlement in the Halford case, the Home Office undertook to review the selection procedures for the appointment of senior officers, in consultation with the local authority associations and the Association of Chief Police Officers (ACPO). Around the same time, it was reported that six police forces were taking part in a pilot scheme on part-time working and that the Police Regulations had been changed to allow part-time working in all specializations up to the rank of Superintendent (Equal Opportunities Review 1992 No. 45). There was, however, a distinctly lukewarm response to these initiatives, with evidence that sex discrimination complaints were being deliberately delayed until the time limits for filing industrial tribunal applications had expired and at least one force failed to issue its officers with the new Home Office circular on part-time working (*The Times*, 7 February 1994).

Women officers were being penalized both ways, denied the opportunity to work part-time where their domestic commitments required it, and yet stereotyped as unsuited to the full responsibilities of police work for reasons of their biology. On returning to work as a police indexer after having had her baby, Sheila Burgess had made childcare arrangements which would ensure that she could resume her old job, including working overtime. In fact, her overtime virtually disappeared, which caused her severe financial difficulties. When the case was heard, her superior officers stated that they had assumed that she had childcare problems, despite her denials. The tribunal accepted the employer's arguments; Sheila Burgess became ill through depression, believing that she would from then on be regarded as a troublemaker, and the police force lost the services of a first class indexer (Radio 4 *World Tonight Special*, 26 September 1996).

In 1994, the first woman was appointed to the rank for which Alison Halford's superiors had refused to consider her, that of Deputy Chief Constable. Elizabeth Neville became the highest ranking operational policewoman when she was appointed DCC of Northamptonshire. One year later, Pauline Clare became Britain's first woman Chief Constable, appointed to head the Lancashire force. The rank of DCC, along with the rank of Chief Superintendent, has since been abolished in England and Wales and Ms Neville has been promoted to the post of Chief Constable of Wiltshire. By 1997, there were still only nine women members of the ACPO compared with some 250 men. Despite all the recruitment drives, women still represent only 14 per cent of the total force and are concentrated at the bottom of the hierarchy. Although 17 per cent of police constables are women, the percentages then drop dramatically, so that only 6 per cent of sergeants, 4 per cent of inspectors and chief inspectors and 3 per cent of superintendents are women (EOC 1997).

A report by Her Majesty's Inspectorate of Constabulary (HMIC) published in 1992 confirmed that the cult of masculinity was still flourishing and that women were seriously under-represented in mainstream Criminal Investigation Departments (CID), traffic and training posts and over-represented in community relations and juvenile posts. The inspection found evidence from sickness records, from interviews with police medical officers and from policewomen themselves that they were suffering persistent low-level harassment unchecked by supervisors (HMIC 1992). A second report published in 1996 was no less critical: 'Alongside praiseworthy examples of good practice, there is also scepticism, tokenism and indifference' (HMIC 1996: 9). The report found slow progress up the promotion ladder for women and ethnic minorities, alongside continuing high levels of sexist and racist banter and harassment and discrimination against civilian staff.

> All too often this behaviour went unchallenged by peers and superiors. Many women and ethnic minority staff felt that anyone who raised issues would be denigrated, ignored or dealt with inappropriately, and most had developed coping mechanisms in order to continue with work which they valued highly. There were comments about a perceived lack of top-level commitment to equal opportunities and its effect on middle management.
>
> (HMIC 1996: 9)

The report makes it clear that equal opportunities is not a 'bolt-on soft option' but is essential for 'the creation of a Service grounded in fairness in which every member, irrespective of gender, race, sexual orientation, disability or background, can flourish, develop and give of their best' (ibid. 10).

It seems pertinent to ask just how many critical reports and tribunal cases are going to be required before there is tangible evidence of improvement. The EOC has expressed its exasperation:

> It is just extraordinary that they have all these equal opportunities policies and yet they are not following them through. It is not beneficial to the women. It is not beneficial to the men or their employer.
>
> (*Daily Telegraph*, 23 February 1996)

The EOC believes that women make good police officers and good community officers so that managers like to hang on to them; they also need them to search women criminals. This means that they tend not to encourage them to join specialist units or seek promotion. The important issue, according to the EOC, is to get the women into the specialist units such as firearms, the royal protection squad, dog handling and the mounted police and to ensure that they are there in groups of four or five so that they are not isolated (private communication, EOC). If this goal is to be achieved, it will obviously require a change of heart on the part of local managers, who will need to encourage the women to apply for specialist training. It will also require a careful scrutiny of the working conditions within the specialist units; if these are not congenial the women will simply leave and the training will be wasted.

This same theme was explored on the eve of the Police Federation conference in Blackpool in May 1997, when two senior policewomen expressed their concern that although some 30 per cent of new recruits were women, few managed to achieve promotion or gain admission to specialist areas such as the firearm squads. They believed that the women were often hesitant to apply for specialist posts, partly because of the irregular hours and partly in case they found themselves the sole woman in an otherwise all male unit. A woman firearms officer from Essex confirmed that there were fewer women firearms officers in her force than had been the case in 1977 (*Guardian*, 20 May 1997).

In March 1997, an industrial tribunal heard of the resentment that is engendered when a woman officer dares to be too successful. Cydena Fleming, an inspector with the Lincolnshire Police Force, had been commended in a Police Promotions Board report for her 'exceptional level of performance', her strength of character, communication skills, first class brain and abundance of enthusiasm. Within months of receiving such a glowing endorsement, Inspector Fleming was being subjected to unrelenting abuse and animosity as her male colleagues attempted to force her out. Reluctantly, she complained about the obsessive behaviour of one particular officer, but received no help from her superiors. Her lawyer described to the tribunal how her career had been destroyed by a combination of sexual harassment and institutional hostility (*Daily Telegraph*, 4 March 1997)

When senior officers refused to take her complaint seriously, Cydena Fleming placed a tape recorder in her locker to obtain evidence of the harassment; the discovery of this action led to her suspension. Giving full support to the junior officers who had made her life a misery and had also broken into her locker, her superiors directed the full weight of disciplinary proceedings exclusively against her. Inspector Fleming therefore had to seek a remedy outside the force and so used the industrial tribunal system to lodge a complaint of sex discrimination and victimization. The tribunal hearing lasted 63 days and involved 72 witnesses; running in parallel with the case, the Humberside force was brought in to conduct an inquiry into events in Lincolnshire. Eventually, in February 1998 an industrial tribunal upheld Cydena Fleming's charge of victimization and in June the Lincolnshire force offered her an apology and an undisclosed sum by way of compensation.

It is difficult to estimate the negative impact of this case, in terms of damaged careers, adverse publicity, misuse of police time and financial cost (the legal costs alone incurred by the Lincolnshire force amounted to some £350,000). All of this could have been avoided if senior officers had treated the initial complaint seriously and conducted their own internal investigation into the matters raised.

## Sexual and racial harassment

The celebrated case of Police Constable Sarah Locker serves to highlight many of the issues raised in this chapter: the existence of a sexist and racist 'cop culture' within the police; the structural and cultural obstacles that prevent female and ethnic minority officers from career progression; the tendency of the police to react defensively and then, having belatedly admitted liability, to attempt yet again to put their house in order.

Sarah Locker joined the Metropolitan Police in 1980 and made an excellent start, receiving four commendations in just a few years. Even so, her applications to transfer to the Criminal Investigation Department were turned down and male colleagues with shorter periods of service were promoted ahead of her. She claimed that pornographic magazines were left on her desk and that she was subjected to racial abuse. After she filed her tribunal application for sex and race discrimination, she found that fellow officers refused to speak to her and threats were made against her. One of WPC Locker's complaints was that because of her Turkish origins, the police had been pleased to use her services as an interpreter on numerous occasions, but had then used this against her when she had applied for promotion, arguing that she had spent too much time away from operational duties (Equal Opportunities Review (1994) No. 53: 8).

The case was supported by the Equal Opportunities Commission and the Commission for Racial Equality. WPC Locker was initially offered the derisory sum of £250 to settle the case. Two and a half years later, the Metropolitan Police agreed to settle for the sum of £25,000 plus £7,500 towards the legal costs; the Police Commissioner and the alleged harasser both apologized and the Commissioner undertook to review certain aspects of the Met.'s equal opportunities policies. The agreement also included arrangements for Sarah Locker to continue her career within the police, including provision for CID training and for a senior woman detective to act as mentor, but in fact she had had enough and retired on medical grounds. Sarah described how she was subjected to hours and hours of interrogation late into the night, although she was six months pregnant at the time (Radio 4 *World Tonight Special*, 26 September 1996). Although the grievance procedure has since been made less arduous, there is still an enormous amount of resentment if an officer 'breaks ranks' and tells tales on her colleagues.

Paradoxically, as some aspects of equal opportunities policies have begun to take effect, with the recruitment of more women and even the promotion of a small number to senior positions, resentment on the part of many male officers has evidently increased. This backlash would come as no surprise to Francis Heidensohn, who believes that policemen are fully aware of the fraudulent nature of their macho characterization of police work, but that the central issue is 'the gendered claim to sole ownership of the rights to social control' (Heidensohn 1992: 14). Clearly, it is not simply a gendered claim, as Heidensohn herself acknowledges, as other groups are also excluded from the 'cop culture', notably police men and women who are members of minority racial and ethnic groups. Holdaway gives a very moving account of how black and Asian officers become worn down by the continual use of racist language, whether it was directed at them or not. As one officer explained:

They make you realise that you are not the same as them. You are
not an officer first – to them you are an Asian officer....You are an
Asian person and then an officer.

(Holdaway 1996: 163)

There is growing evidence of a rising incidence of bullying within
police forces, particularly an increase in sexist and racist banter.
Sharon Parker found that one in eight of the women employed by the
South Yorkshire Police had experienced unwelcome touching. She
believes that women officers cope better than men with the routine
aspects of police work and that they are better at interacting with the
community. The bullying and harassment are therefore often expressions of jealousy (Radio 4 *World Tonight Special* 1996). There can be
no doubt that complaints of sexual and racial harassment by police
women and men are on the increase. This can be attributed both to the
backlash against equal opportunities policies from within the operational ranks and to the greater willingness of police officers on the
receiving end of such harassment to come forward.

Even so, the cases that are reported are merely the tip of the iceberg.
The vast majority of women struggle on in silence, aware of the
hostility that awaits them if they dare to 'rock the boat', doubtful that
they will be supported by senior officers and certain that their long-
term career prospects within the police will be irreparably damaged.
Like Sarah Locker, those women who do report harassment usually do
so when they have reached the end of the road and abandoned the idea
of remaining in the force.

Another officer interviewed in the Radio 4 programme 'Can't you
take a joke?' only spoke out about her experiences after she had retired
from the force due to an injury at work. She described how she had
entered into the spirit of the practical jokes, accepting them as harmless fun, but when she began working with a new team, the jokes took a
sinister turn. They involved crude nicknames being shouted across the
station, male officers boasting about their sexual conquests, including
buggering a woman and tying her up when drunk, the exchange of
pornographic pictures and the officer herself being forced to bend over
while they stamped the name of the police station on her backside and
then held her down for simulated sex. She put up with abuse for years,
because her boss warned her that if she complained she would be put
back in uniform (Radio 4 *World Tonight Special* 1996).

This officer recognized that she was trapped in a male culture that
disapproved strongly of anyone who broke ranks and blew the whistle
on colleagues. This is confirmed by the experience of a male officer

who had unusually broken ranks in order to appear as a witness in a sexual harassment case, giving evidence in support of the complainant. Assuming that he must be having an affair with the woman concerned, his colleagues extended the harassment to him and his superiors began a close scrutiny of his work. Suffering from headaches, insomnia and marital problems because of this persecution, the officer described harassment as a dripping tap that slowly destroys the working environment (Radio 4 *World Tonight Special* 1996).

It is the acceptance by policemen of persistent low-level harassment as a normal part of the everyday working environment that creates the conditions within which serious sexual attacks are likely to occur. In 1993, Tina Martin and Lyn Coles of the British Association of Women Police, operating an informal counselling service and receiving around 12 calls a week, made the following comment to Janet Cohen:

> We have examples of women who will go into their inspector's office only in pairs, right up to a woman who's been raped while on duty in a police station. They are otherwise assertive women who are reduced to quivering wrecks.
>
> (Cohen 1993)

Where the women are not totally isolated and other female officers in the same unit or police station are experiencing similar treatment, they may well be able to find strength in acting collectively, particularly where senior officers are condoning or turning a blind eye to the harassment, or even initiating it themselves. Janet Cohen spoke to a group of women who discovered that they were all being harassed by the same inspector, so they decided to lodge an official complaint. The Assistant Chief Constable took the complaint so seriously that he decided to bypass the grievance procedure in favour of a criminal prosecution for indecent assault. The Director of Public Prosecutions decided that a prosecution would not be in the public interest and the case was dropped. Although the inspector was transferred to another position, his career is seemingly intact and the women officers are left disillusioned, the hope of an effective remedy snatched away from them (Cohen 1993).

The lack of a clear and consistent policy within the police on how to deal with sexual harassment is epitomized by the case of Karen Wade. She lost the tribunal case in which she complained of sexual harassment by three of her male colleagues, not least because the police pleaded Public Interest Immunity which prevented documents used during the internal investigation from being made available to the tribunal. The Police Federation decided to represent the three male officers in this case, so that Karen was represented by an unqualified relative. Despite this outcome, Chief Constable Keith Hellawell decided that action was needed to curb the excess of 'laddishness' in the West Yorkshire force and the clique of officers who had worked with Karen Wade was broken up. Monitoring systems were put in place, with the result that disciplinary action has been taken against a number of officers. On appeal, the Public Interest Immunity was lifted and Karen Wade will now be able to tell the whole story to the tribunal (Radio 4 *World Tonight Special* 1996).

When it comes to pursuing their attackers through the courts, an additional factor that may well deter women officers is their inside knowledge of the traumas suffered by women in general who report rape to the police and also the extremely low chances of securing a conviction. One might expect women officers to be accepted as credible, articulate and reliable witnesses, thereby increasing the chances of a successful outcome, but the few cases that come to court provide no evidence that this is so.

In February 1988 a women police constable claimed that she was buggered and raped by a colleague in her room in a police section house in the early hours of the morning. Both of them were off-duty at the time. WPC Waters alleged she had later discovered that her virginity had been the topic of conversation at a police drinking session, a bottle of whisky had been wagered and a senior officer had driven her assailant to the section house (Toolis 1993). When Eileen Waters reported the rape, she was transferred to another police station and subjected to a gruelling interrogation by two Police Federation officials. Following an internal inquiry by a detective superintendent, no action was taken against the male officer. Eileen Waters states that from then on, she was ostracized, a campaign of petty harassment was waged against her and her career ground to a halt; also that her name was removed from the list of specially trained officers used for police searches.

Having in her view been let down so badly by the internal grievance procedures, she filed a tribunal application for victimization under the Sex Discrimination Act, linking it to her allegation of sexual assault. The tribunal dismissed the complaint on the grounds that the alleged acts were not committed by the police officer in the course of his employment and so her employer, the Commissioner of the Metropolitan Police, could not be held liable. This decision was upheld by the Employment Appeal Tribunal (Equal Opportunities Review 1995 No. 64: 40), so that the legal system also failed WPC Waters. The worst aspect of her experience was the vicious sexism she encountered at every level within the Metropolitan Police command structure....From the outset, [her] superiors viewed her allegation not as a report of a criminal offence but as a threat to the reputation of the Metropolitan Police that had to be neutralised.

(Toolis 1993: 8 and 10)

It can be of no consolation to the Metropolitan Police that Eileen Waters lost her case on legal grounds without the facts being considered, particularly as a similar case of racial harassment (not against the police), heard by the Employment Appeal Tribunal at the same time and dismissed on these grounds, was reversed on appeal by the Court of Appeal. The legal arguments centred on the meaning of the phrase 'in the course of employment'. The judges recognized that if the phrase were to be interpreted narrowly in accordance with tort law principles, it would have the paradoxical effect that 'the more heinous the act of discrimination, the less likely it will be that the employer would be liable' (*Jones* v. *Tower Boot Co Ltd* [1977] IRLR 168). Rejecting this approach, the Court opted for a commonsense interpretation of the phrase 'in the course of employment'.

Eileen Waters had also pursued a civil action against the Police Commissioner for negligence, seeking damages and an injunction, restraining him and his officers from interfering with her duties as a police officer and from harassment and intimidation. The claim was dismissed by the High Court on the grounds that it disclosed no reasonable cause of action. WPC Waters appealed to the Court of Appeal against both decisions. Dealing with the negligence claim, the Court confirmed the decision of the High Court, holding that the Commissioner had no personal duty of care to a police officer and that there were 'well-established policy reasons' for this situation:

A police officer does not owe a duty of care to another officer. Therefore, the Commissioner was not vicariously liable for torts committed against the appellants by other officers under his direction and control. If other police officers owed the appellant a duty of care, breach of which would render the appellant jointly liable in negligence, it would become necessary for the courts to investigate the internal discipline of the force.

(*Waters* v. *Commissioner of Police of the Metropolis* [1997] IRLR 590)

In relation to the victimization claim, the Court of Appeal was no longer concerned with the strict application of tort law principles in assessing employer liability and, following *Jones* v. *Tower Boot Co Ltd*, were entitled to take a broader view. 'In the course of employment' was to be given the meaning it had in everyday speech (*Jones* v. *Tower Boot Co Ltd*). Unfortunately, the way that the evidence had been presented at the first tribunal hearing meant that it was not possible to argue the employer-liability issue in the way that it should have been argued. Statements of fact agreed by both parties at the outset of the proceedings meant that key questions, such as the alleged complicity of a senior officer in encouraging the assailant to accept a bet to try and 'have' WPC Waters, and the extent to which the police are required to take responsibility for incidents occurring in the section house, could not be raised. An appeal has to be lodged on a point of law, so that factual evidence presented at the tribunal stage cannot be altered for the appeal. The tribunal had approached the issue as a simple case of two work colleagues who developed a sexual relationship outside work. Eileen Waters was left without a remedy either for the alleged rape or the apparent victimization that followed her reporting of the rape. This is difficult to comprehend. Even if the Commissioner insists that he has no responsibility for events occurring in the section house during off duty hours, it is undeniably his responsibility to ensure that officers reporting sexual and racial harassment are not victimized as a result of making these complaints (whether they are eventually substantiated or not) and that all allegations are thoroughly investigated.

In February 1995, PC Michael Seear was acquitted of raping a female colleague after a New Year's Eve party. The woman officer had waited three months before making her complaint. She explained she had hoped to block out what had happened to her and to carry on as normal. She stated that she found this impossible and she became increasingly distressed and began having nightmares. She reported the alleged attack and the case went to a criminal trial rather than an industrial tribunal. It was the first criminal trial involving police officers as both complainant and defendant to reach court. In the absence of any forensic evidence, it was his word against hers; Seear was acquitted and called for the lifting of the anonymity rule so that his accuser could be named. Once again the alleged attack took place in a police section house where the two officers lived. Both of them were probationers and had been good friends until the attack. The policewoman's boyfriend was also a serving police officer living in the same section house and PC Seear's best friend; hence the complainant said, her hesitation and delay in reporting the incident. PC Seear admitted that he had been drinking heavily on the night in question but insisted that the sexual encounter was by mutual consent and had not involved full intercourse.

It is rare for cases involving police officers as both complainant and defendant to reach court, although according to a study by Anderson, Brown and Campbell (1993) of 1,800 policewomen, nearly all had experienced some form of sexual harassment, 30 per cent had experienced unwanted touching or pinching by fellow officers in the six months prior to the study and 6 per cent had suffered serious sexual assault by a male colleague. It is no coincidence that a large proportion of these attacks take place in section houses, where women officers are entering a largely male preserve, where women probationers are particularly vulnerable and where 'men are men and women are Plonks – persons of little or no knowledge' (comment by a female officer, reported in the *Daily Telegraph*, 21 February 1995). Off duty time is spent in heavy drinking, frequent parties and horseplay and the women officers have to find some way of accommodating to this culture. Sexual attacks are rarely reported. Inspector Ana Starcevic, who researched the issue of sexual harassment in the police for her thesis *The Ungentle Touch* (1993) said:

> Imagine reporting a sex offence by a colleague, then having to hand your underwear over for examination to someone on your own force, someone you probably know.
>
> (*Daily Telegraph*, 21 February 1995. See also Starcevic 1995)

Her research was prompted by her own experience of a sexual assault when she was a probationer, an attack which she never reported. For most women officers, reporting an attack marks the end of their careers in the police, but the officer in the Seear case expressed her intention of continuing in the force, devoting her career to counselling rape victims:

> The only way I can see forward is not to let this incident completely mess up my life. I have to use it to say to victims: 'I can understand'.
>
> (*Daily Telegraph*, 21 February 1995)

It is to be hoped that this WPC will not be forced out of the police force as a consequence of her courage in making her complaint and also that the decision by the Surrey police to allow this case to go to trial rather than attempt to sweep it under the carpet indicates a determination by the police to treat all such incidents seriously in the future. This does not necessarily mean that there will be an epidemic of tribunal cases. Most women officers would probably prefer their complaints to be dealt with internally, so long as their accounts are treated seriously and appropriate remedies found. However, since the removal of the ceiling on compensation levels in discrimination cases, the costs of dealing with the aftermath of harassment, rather than preventing its occurrence in the first place, are likely to be high.[2]

In September 1996, North Yorkshire Police made an out of court settlement of more than £110,000 to two women officers who reported sexual harassment from male colleagues. It took four years for the women to come forward, complaining of bullying, bizarre initiation rites, sexist comments and always being given the worst jobs. The terms of the settlement included an agreement by the women not to talk about the case, but the father of one of them commented: 'She has a number of commendations from the force, including one for bravery after she disarmed a man in a hostage situation'. He expressed the view that the culture of sexual harassment and bullying was so pervasive that senior officers must have been aware of what was going on; if they were not aware, there was something seriously wrong with the force (*The Times*, 18 September 1996).

Sixteen months later, the aftershock from this case was still reverberating throughout the North Yorkshire force as a series of internal inquiries and appeals, all subject to the Home Office rules on public interest immunity, became bogged down in what one journalist described as 'near farce' (*Guardian*, 9 January 1998). With the Chief Constable facing disciplinary action, the local MP attempted to penetrate the wall of secrecy surrounding the case. Describing legal rules governing the report prepared by the Chief Constable of Nottinghamshire as more akin to Stalinist Russia than late twentieth century Britain, he also commented on the secrecy surrounding reports prepared by his local police authority: 'When the reports contain details of alleged misconduct and payment of hundreds of thousands of pounds and questions the operational ability of the chief constable, then the public has a right to know' (Paul Willis MP, quoted in the *Guardian*, 9 January 1998).

In all the early cases involving complaints of sexual harassment by policewomen, either the tribunal found against the complainant or the case was settled at some point in the proceedings, prior to the tribunal reaching a decision. In the very first case to be decided in favour of a policewoman harassed by a male colleague, the definition of 'in the course of employment' in determining employer liability for the behaviour of employees was reconsidered. The case of *Stubbs* v. *the Chief Constable of Lincolnshire and Detective Sergeant Walker*, heard in July 1997, lasted fourteen days with the applicant calling three witnesses and the respondents twenty-three (Case No. 38395/96). Detective Constable Stubbs complained of sexual harassment and sex discrimination. She had been making steady progress in her career until she joined the Regional Crime Squad and encountered Detective Sergeant Walker. He had made a play for her sexually and when she had rejected his advances, he began treating her in an abusive and hostile manner, giving her a bad appraisal report and excluding her from an important surveillance operation.

DC Stubbs was the only woman on her team, a situation she had also faced in her previous position on the Lincolnshire Drug Squad; she was also the first woman officer to complete an extremely demanding covert rural surveillance course. Early reports had described her as reliable and conscientious with a flair for surveillance operations, so that the adverse report from DS Walker stood in sharp contradiction to all prior assessments of her work. Even so, her superior officers failed to take her complaint seriously and also refused to acknowledge that the only plausible explanation for the adverse report was that DS Walker was taking his revenge. Despite the large number of witnesses paraded before them on the respondent's side as the police closed ranks against the complainant, the tribunal found the evidence of DC Stubbs to be the most credible. Fortunately, she had kept a careful record of the key events in a notebook, on the advice of a policewoman friend and confidante. She had also told her doctor about the harassment, as she began suffering from symptoms of depression, including sleeplessness, weeping and loss of appetite.

The tribunal found the evidence of DS Walker unconvincing and his attitudes sexist; they also concluded that the evidence provided by his work colleagues was motivated by ill-will and prejudice. It was clear to the tribunal that the detective chief inspector who had investigated DC Stubbs' complaint had failed to take the matter seriously. When the Chief Constable became involved, he too refused to accept that the most likely explanation for the bad appraisal report was sex discrimination. It is astonishing that the police allowed this case to go so far, thereby tying up a great deal of police time, with so many officers appearing before the tribunal. Perhaps a degree of complacency had set in, following 'successes' in earlier cases, as complainants failed to convince tribunals of the merits of their cases. Perhaps it is a lack of familiarity with the standard of proof in civil cases, decided on the balance of probabilities, rather than in accordance with the criminal standard of adjudication, 'beyond reasonable doubt'.

In any event, it will be important for the police to take note of the tribunal's findings on employer liability, particularly in relation to the definition of 'in the course of employment'. Following the earlier ruling in *Jones* v. *Tower Boot* that tribunals should adopt a common-sense interpretation of this phrase, the tribunal refers to two incidents of harassment and abuse that occurred outside working time and concludes that: 'Attending a public house for relaxation immediately after the end of the working day is, in our view, merely an extension of employment' (*Stubbs* v. *the Chief Constable of Lincolnshire and Detective Sergeant Walker*: 12) and similarly that attending a leaving party for a work colleague 'is an extension of work and the workplace' (ibid. 14). Adopting a very different approach from that taken in the Waters' case, the tribunal holds that:

> Work related social functions are an extension of employment and we can see no reason to restrict the course of employment purely to what goes on in the workplace.
>
> (*Stubbs* v. *the Chief Constable of Lincolnshire and Detective Sergeant Walker*: 29)

This decision is the subject of an appeal, the outcome of which will have profound implications for employer-liability within the police service and in the labour market more generally.

Two months later, WPC Kay Kellaway won her case for sex discrimination and victimization against the Thames Valley Police in a majority tribunal decision. After accusing an officer from another force of sexually assaulting her, Kay Kellaway claimed that she was labelled a 'whore, bitch and slag' by her male colleagues, that her sexuality became the subject of secret reports between senior officers and that pressure was put on her to withdraw her application for promotion. When she was promoted to acting sergeant, she claimed that a Detective Superintendent referred to her as 'taking jobs from the boys' (*Guardian*, 24 September 1997). When she joined the force, she had been considered a model officer and during her probationary period came first out of 32 officers. Early reports noted that she was a determined, self-motivated officer who required a minimum of supervision. Then she discovered by chance that the same DS who had made it clear that he did not approve of policewomen had added some highly derogatory remarks to her personal file. She told the tribunal that none of the points made had been discussed with her and since then several documents had mysteriously disappeared. Thames Valley's insistence that it has done more than any other comparable force to promote women to senior ranks and to ensure that career structures are free from discrimination (ibid.) merely draws attention to the continuing

gap between policy statements emanating from the top and the continuing resistance of many middle-ranking and some senior police
officers to their effective implementation. Thames Valley Police have
lodged an appeal against the tribunal decision in this case.

In November 1997, the Thames Valley Police were in the news again,
when Detective Constable Dee Mazurkiewicz won her case for sexual
harassment. She told the tribunal how her colleagues had nicknamed
her 'WDC Massive Cleavage' and spread rumours that she persuaded
suspects to confess by showing them her breasts and that she gave
sexual favours to informants. In reply to these allegations, it was argued
that WDC Mazurkiewicz had herself participated in sexist jokes and
that male officers also had derogatory nicknames; the examples given
were 'Bonky', 'Porky' and 'Gonzo' (Duncan Campbell 1997).

Such a line of defence does occasionally prove successful in sex
discrimination cases, as it is necessary for the complainant to prove
that she (or he) has received less favourable treatment than a person of
the opposite sex would receive and that this constitutes a detriment
(Sex Discrimination Act 1975 sections 1 and 6). For example, if it can
be shown that displays of pornographic material were such that men as
well as women might have found them offensive, it could be argued
that no discrimination has occurred.[3] Fortunately, most industrial
tribunals adopt a commonsense approach to such issues and are
increasingly willing to disregard claims that sexist and racist banter is
harmless fun and is neutral in its impact. The fact that Dee
Mazurkiewicz had been on sick leave suffering from stress for almost
three years by the time the case was heard is evidence enough of the
damaging effects of harassment.

The tribunal reached its decision by assessing all the evidence and
finding in favour of the WDC 'on the balance of probabilities'. An
internal inquiry under the police complaints procedure had dismissed
the complaint, applying the higher standard of proof 'beyond reasonable doubt'. ACPO has argued for a lowering of the standard of proof
in cases involving police discipline, whereas the Police Federation
wishes to retain the status quo. The Thames Valley Police were so
concerned about the adverse publicity surrounding this case that they
produced a forty-page press pack outlining their equal opportunities
policies and their commitment to women officers. Despite strenuous
efforts to recruit and promote women and to stamp out boorish
behaviour, the Thames Valley Police, along with the rest of the police
service, are likely to find themselves on the receiving end of similar
cases in the future. It is essential that internal mechanisms are put in

place to deal with all complaints of harassment swiftly and effectively, and so minimize the chances of more cases occurring in the future.

## Male-dominated workplaces: a danger zone for women

The police service is not alone in facing problems of harassment within its workforce. Bullying and harassment at work is a long-standing and widespread phenomenon, although recognition of its damaging consequences and the creation of policies designed to address it are relatively new. For a long time, sexual harassment was accepted by both men and women as an inevitable consequence of women moving into the public sphere, a constant reminder to women that they were encroaching on male terrain and could expect to be treated first and foremost as sexual beings and only secondarily as workers. Such treatment was clearly incompatible with the spirit and intention of the Sex Discrimination Act and gradually industrial tribunals came to recognize that sexual harassment did constitute 'less favourable treatment' and a 'detriment' under the terms of the Act, although the term sexual harassment did not actually appear in the legislation (Gregory 1995). Nowadays, with the additional force of European law underpinning the domestic legislation, most employers have adopted policies and grievance procedures as an insurance against expensive litigation.

Sexual harassment takes a variety of forms, but it is important to recognize that it is part of the continuum of male violence against women. It often assumes its most threatening and dangerous form where women are trying to break into male-dominated areas of work. For example, British Rail began to call itself 'an equal opportunities employer' in the early 1980s, but in fact only 6 per cent of the workers were women, working mainly as secretaries, cleaners and canteen staff. A research report published in 1986 showed that these women suffered the usual lack of career progression and sexist teasing common in many female servicing roles, where running errands and flattering male egos becomes an integral part of their daily tasks. The really vicious forms of harassment were reserved for the women trainee drivers, including graffiti, anonymous letters and daily abuse:

> Some days the mess-room may be full of pornography 'that looks as if it came out of a gynaecological text-book'. Women may be touched, insulted, pushed and threatened: 'one driver goes a little bit further each time'. They can report the offender and increase

their unpopularity; or they can put up with it until the situation at
work begins to colour everything they do.

(Robbins 1986: 57)

The London Fire Brigade, where the Greater London Council
(GLC) had taken positive steps to recruit women and ethnic minority
men and women into the fire service, experienced a similar reaction
from their existing workforce. Firefighter Lynne Gunning complained
of sexual harassment alleging that her male colleagues tied her to a
ladder, hosed her down with water, subjected her to sexual abuse and
indecently exposed themselves to her. It was also alleged that she had
urine poured over her, and all of this was dismissed by other firemen
as a bizarre but harmless initiation ceremony. As seven men were
suspended from duty pending an official inquiry, 7,000 firemen threatened to strike if any of the accused men were dismissed (*Daily
Telegraph*, 20 July 1984). One firefighter was dismissed but subsequently reinstated on appeal to the GLC Public Services and Fire
Brigade Committee.

Male-dominated organizations which require their employees to
spend at least part of their working time operating in dangerous conditions, as is the case in the fire brigade, the police force and the armed
services, face particular difficulties. The bonding that takes place
between the men could be regarded as an inevitable and beneficial
feature of their working conditions; there has to be mutual trust and
co-operation in situations of danger. Unfortunately, the downside of
this male bonding is that it excludes anyone not accepted as part of the
in-group. It is easier to treat women and ethnic minority colleagues as
outsiders, reinforcing the group culture by making them the butt of
sexist and racist jokes, rather than shift the group norms so as to
accommodate the newcomers within the group.

The presenter of the ITV *World in Action* programme 'Conduct
Unbecoming' (1997) asked 'Why does a uniform make men behave
badly?'. This may be the wrong way to pose the question, but the
programme did provide evidence that sexual harassment is still deeply
embedded within our uniformed services. Tania Clayton claimed that
while serving as a firefighter, she was ordered to cut her hair although
it was already shorter than that of some of the men; that she was never
allowed to make any mistakes during training, unlike the men, and
that on the nightshift, she even found herself getting up half an hour
earlier than everyone else, in order to take her workmates tea in bed!
She described how her confidence became so eroded that she ceased to
function properly. Matters came to a head when one officer put her in

a cage 100 feet in the air and spun her around for an hour, ostensibly to cure her (non-existent) fear of heights. In 1997, an industrial tribunal awarded her an apology and £200,000 in compensation.

Also in 1997, the first woman officer to sue the army for sexual harassment won an apology and an out of court settlement. As a result of a 'gagging clause' included in the agreement, the details of the settlement are not known, but Alisa Cook told an earlier tribunal how male officers who resented her promotion had subjected her to a barrage of sexual innuendo. On one occasion she said, they locked her in a shower room and gassed her with CS pellets (*Express*, 22 February 1997). She described to the *World in Action* interviewer just how close she had come to throwing herself out of the third storey window. In another case, Lisa Nicholson was also paid off by the army and subjected to a gagging order; there are more cases in the pipeline. One sergeant committed suicide before allegations of rape made against him could be investigated. On behalf of the army, Brigadier Andrew Cumming regretted the delays in investigating complaints, attributing these to the small size of the army investigation branch. More positively, he spoke of the new measures that were being introduced, including a bullying helpline and harassment awareness training (*World in Action* 1997).

The opening scenes of the *World in Action* programme showed Bernard Manning telling sexist and racist jokes at a social event organized on behalf of the Manchester police. It seems extraordinary that such an event could have been permitted, especially as Bernard Manning's grotesque sense of humour had been the subject of an earlier tribunal case, in which the management of the hotel hosting the event at which he was speaking were found to be liable for failing to protect two black waitresses from racial harassment by Mr Manning and other dinner guests. (*Burton and Rhule* v. *De Vere Hotels* [1996] IRLR 596)

Despite the reassurances given on *World in Action* by Chief Constable Tony Burden of the ACPO Equal Opportunities Committee, that there was a one hundred per cent commitment on the part of the police force to ensure fairness throughout the service, and that anyone found guilty of sexual harassment would be sacked, it has yet to be demonstrated that any of the uniformed services have the problem of harassment firmly under control. The firefighters who tormented Tania Clayton were given nothing more than a verbal warning. Sarah Locker, who described life inside the police station as more threatening than life on the street, asked why it was that most of the women who made complaints no longer had a job in the police service, whereas some of the men may have been moved but their long-term careers are seemingly undamaged (*World in Action* 1997).

Research confirms that certain features of organizations increase the chances of gender stereotyping, so that sexualized behaviour towards women is normalized as part of the occupational culture. These characteristics include women forming less than 20 per cent of the organization, women working alone in particular locations, and the availability of sexually explicit material (Brown *et al.* 1995). All these characteristics apply to the police, including the presence of explicit materials related to sexual crimes. Significantly, Brown *et al.* find that civilian women working within the police environment are less likely to be exposed to harassment than women police officers. Although this is due in part to the fact that 60 per cent of the total civilian staff are female and that they tend to be slightly older on average than the women officers, it can also be explained in terms of the support, administrative and secretarial work that they do, work which does not directly challenge the gender stereotypes. Brown *et al.* conclude that:

> the differential rates of sexual harassment between civilian and police women...are a function of the threat posed to police men's occupational identity by women's incursion into their male preserves.
>
> (Brown *et al.* 1995: 227)

They also found that policewomen were more likely to focus on frustrated career progression than on their experiences of harassment as an explanation for any problems they were encountering, and yet it was clear from the responses to the General Health Questionnaire, completed by the officers who participated in the study, that sexual harassment was the better predictor of psychological distress. The researchers' explanation for this is that concerns about lack of career progress are more acceptable; that it is still countercultural to blow the whistle on a colleague by complaining about his behaviour. They emphasize the importance of uncovering the hidden phenomenon of the non-reporting and under-reporting of sexual harassment (Brown *et al.* 1995).

## Conclusion

The cases described in this chapter represent a small selection from those appearing in the law reports or highlighted by the media in recent years. In view of the difficulties in obtaining official material or conducting research on the issues raised in this chapter, it has proved necessary to pull together information from a variety of sources. The survey data which is available (see for example Anderson *et al.* 1993, Brown 1998) confirms the problem of harassment is widespread and endemic, a cancer which is eating away at the morale of the force and proving extremely costly both in terms of wasted careers and financial compensation. It is bound to affect the quality of service delivery that police forces can provide, partly because they are losing precisely those officers who are best equipped to deal sympathetically and effectively with complainants in rape and sexual assault cases, but also because it damages their public image and undermines their credibility. As Peter Moorhouse, Chair of the Police Complaints Authority put it:

> There is certainly a perception within the public mind that if the police service is unable to manage sexual and racial relationships between officers, what hope is there that such relationships will be well managed by individual officers in their day-to-day contacts with members of the public.
>
> (*Guardian*, 4 July 1997)

In other parts of the labour market, the trade unions have played an important role in the fight against sexual and racial harassment. Abandoning their earlier stance that they were reluctant to take sides when both the complainant and the harasser were union members, they now have a clear policy that harassment is unacceptable behaviour in the workplace. In the early 1980s the Trades Union Congress produced a Black Workers Charter (TUC 1981) and guidelines on Sexual Harassment at Work (TUC 1983). Although there was no overnight transformation, and sexual and racial harassment have by no means been eliminated from the workplace, at least complainants who were members of trade unions had somewhere they could turn for support. The Police Federation has yet to resolve the dilemma that its membership includes officers complaining of harassment and officers accused of harassment, and that both groups are likely to seek support from the Federation. In the meantime, women and ethnic minority officers are beginning to raise the profile of this issue in a variety of ways.

The fifteen most senior women in the Metropolitan Police, those at the level of chief inspector or above, have formed an advisory group to raise awareness of the problems women officers face. They believe that the present assessment process constitutes a major deterrent to women considering putting themselves forward for promotion, partly because most of the assessors are men and partly because they fear being isolated as senior officers, because of their small numbers. This is clearly a vicious circle, which can only be broken by promoting a 'critical mass' of women. Anne McDaid, Chief Inspector, police personnel management says:

> The problem for women is their comparative voicelessness. They communicate in different ways from men, but this is not understood by male colleagues. They also find it hard to raise difficult issues for fear of being branded feminists.
>
> (Pickard 1995: 24)

The group of fifteen is pushing for the views of women officers to be taken into account by policy-making bodies.

Various networking groups are emerging as women officers seek strength in mutual support. One of these groups was based at Bramshill, the police staff college, and subsequently moved to the West Midlands Police. It offers confidential advice to women and ethnic minority officers who have experienced discrimination; networking is now being used as a key strategy for overcoming isolation and confronting discriminatory practices (Pickard 1995). Similar considerations had inspired the launching of the Black Police Association in September 1994 by a group of officers in the Metropolitan Police Service. Its aim is to improve the working environment of black members of staff within the Met. It also seeks to provide a support and social network, promote equal opportunities, improve relations between the Met. and black Londoners, and improve recruitment and reduce wastage of black officers (Equal Opportunities Review 1994 No. 58). The Lesbian and Gay Police Association predates both of these initiatives; formed during 1990, it constituted an open challenge to the heterosexual foundations of police culture. In the past, lesbian and gay officers had mainly kept their sexual identities hidden, employing a variety of strategies (Burke 1993). The creation of an association to provide support and advice was an expression of group confidence on the part of some lesbian and gay officers, who made the difficult decision to 'come out' and confront homophobia within the force head on.

As women, ethnic minority men and women, and lesbian and gay officers begin to challenge discriminatory working practices rather than suffer in silence, the number of complaints against individual police officers is likely to rise. Commissioner Paul Condon has referred to the need to root out corruption in the police force, believing that he is dealing with a small minority of officers. When it comes to rooting out sexual and racial harassment, however, there is no evidence that this problem is confined to a small minority. Senior officers can no longer bury their heads in the sand or rely on damage limitation after the event. If they are to stem the flow of complaints, avoid losing competent officers and paying considerable sums of money by way of compensation, they have to act decisively and proactively to stamp out discrimination and harassment before the harm is inflicted. This may involve disciplining, transferring or even dismissing male officers where complaints are substantiated.

Shredding vital documents or hiding behind spurious claims of national security when cases do come to court is at best a delaying tactic and at worst creates the impression that the police have something to hide. In the Stubbs case, the tribunal were able to hear evidence relating to the content of the covert rural surveillance course in private so that sensitive operational information did not reach the public domain. In the Wade case, now that the Public Interest Immunity has been lifted, a similar strategy can be adopted if there is a genuine need for a confidential setting. There cannot be a blanket immunity for the police which automatically supersedes an individual's right to challenge discriminatory treatment. It is essential that the police succeed in recruiting and retaining more women and ethnic minority officers, in order to reduce wastage and raise morale, while at the same time improving the quality of their service delivery and their credibility rating in the eyes of the public.

# 3  Understanding attrition

As we have seen, the police have been subjected to a great deal of critical scrutiny in recent years. They have been under attack for poor service delivery and bad employment practices, particularly in relation to women and minority ethnic groups. Damning criticism has emanated from a number of sources, including official bodies, such as the Women's National Commission, the Equal Opportunities Commission, and Her Majesty's Inspectorate of Constabulary, and from the findings of both Home Office and independent research projects. Attempts to address the issues that recur in report after report have so far met with only partial success, which constitutes a dilemma for senior officers. On the one hand, they are anxious to demonstrate they have responded to the criticisms and that new policies and practices are now working well; on the other hand, further research opens up the possibility of yet another damning report.

Our research project was supported by Islington Council's Police and Crime Prevention Unit, with funding obtained through the Department of the Environment's Inner Cities Programme. It was with the official backing of the Unit that we initially approached local police stations during 1989, with a view to undertaking research to evaluate police practices in relation to crimes of rape and sexual assault. We were fortunate enough to be put in touch with a woman deputy chief superintendent at Holloway police station who was extremely supportive; the chief superintendent at Kings Cross was much more hesitant, pointing out that it was illegal for us to have access to police records. It became apparent that he was genuinely concerned that the high levels of prostitution in the Kings Cross area would distort the research findings in a way that would reflect badly on his station. We also had to clear the research with Scotland Yard and this proved to be even more difficult. The initial response was that we would have to delay the research for at least one year, until another project (Adler 1991) had been completed. By the time this period had elapsed, the deputy chief superintendent was on sick leave and a new chief superintendent had been appointed at Holloway. He withdrew the access to police records which we had previously negotiated.

Although we had appointed a researcher to start work on the project, several more months of difficult negotiation were needed with the chief superintendents at both Holloway and Kings Cross before a compromise was agreed. The police were anxious that they alone should not be required to shoulder the blame for any shortcomings in the system, and we were able to assure them that we were interested in examining multi-agency responses to the problem of sexual assault. An agreement to that effect was signed by all parties. It was also agreed that two women police officers would be seconded to obtain information from the police records; we therefore drew up a detailed list of the information we required (see Appendix). We had certain reservations about this arrangement, as we would have no way of telling whether data was being withheld for some reason, perhaps in order to present the police in a more favourable light. In the event, however, due to the commitment and enthusiasm of the WPCs who were seconded to this task, we were able to obtain better quality information than if we had been given permission to search the records ourselves. Many record forms, especially when cases are ongoing, are not filed but have to be tracked down and may even be held in a different police station. A combination of determination, inside knowledge and personal contacts enabled the women officers to achieve a much higher success rate in the data collection than we could ever have hoped to achieve. In response to our requests, they collated crime report forms held at Holloway and Kings Cross police stations relating to a two year period (September 1988 to September 1990) and presented us with detailed information on 301 reported cases of rape and sexual assault. This method of collecting the data also gave us a more comprehensive picture of 'no criming' than most other studies; research based on the monthly statistical returns to the Home Office will necessarily omit those cases 'no crimed' during the first month, whereas our study includes this information for all reported cases.

Once access had been agreed, we found the police officers whom we dealt with on a daily basis extremely co-operative and committed to the project. Meetings were also held with the two chief superintendents at crucial points in the study; both of whom were now fully supportive of the project. We conducted interviews with a number of officers, including members of the child protection team and the domestic violence units, and police constables and detective inspectors involved in sexual assault cases. The police also sent out a letter on our behalf to complainants, asking if they would be willing to be interviewed as part of the research. We also conducted interviews with various local professional agencies and volunteer groups concerned with issues of sexual assault, including workers from the victim support service specializing in domestic and sexual assault and volunteer workers from a rape crisis centre. Additional information was obtained from an interview with a general practitioner who had a lengthy record of service as a police surgeon, now officially referred to as a forensic medical examiner (FME).

If the police had appeared initially reluctant to participate in the research, gaining access to the Crown Prosecution Service (CPS) was fraught with even more difficulties. A helpful detective inspector had provided us with the telephone number of a woman lawyer working for the CPS, a lawyer who had been involved in a number of sexual assault cases. After one interesting telephone conversation with her, during which she referred to the differences between men and women lawyers in the ways in which they approached such cases, our access to her and the other 'front line' lawyers was effectively blocked by the branch crown prosecutor. He insisted that all requests for assistance were directed through him and, after considerable delay, offered us an interview. He cancelled the first two appointments and attempted to cancel the third, but his letter failed to reach us in time, so we presented ourselves at his offices. At our insistence, the interview did go ahead but the prosecutor chose his words with extreme care, constantly referring to the Code for Crown Prosecutors (1992) and adding very little of significance. He did suggest that if there was any specific information we needed, we should write to him again, but by that time our research was in its final stages and the delaying tactics had proved effective, in so far as we did not pursue this line of inquiry any further.[1]

As a consolation, he did ask the principle law clerk to assist us in identifying a rape case to be heard at the Old Bailey, in case we wished to attend the trial. Ironically, following publication of our research report by Islington Council, the same official, by then responsible for casework decision-making within CPS London, invited us to talk to a senior management conference, attended by branch crown prosecutors and special casework lawyers, about our findings and recommendations in relation to the role of the CPS. Belatedly, he expressed his concern about current decision-making practices in relation to cases of rape and serious sexual assault.

Our research plan had three major objectives: first, to investigate the impact of innovations in police practices on women reporting sexual offences; second, to analyse the rates of attrition (i.e. the process by which cases are dropped), to see whether these had declined as a result of the new policies; third, to assess the role of the CPS and the courts in terms of their impact on service delivery and attrition rates. The findings on service delivery are reported in some detail in Chapters 6 and 7 below. In this chapter and the next, we focus on the processes of attrition.

It was clear from earlier research that the sexual assaults that are reported, whether to a rape crisis centre, a doctor or a police officer, are the mere tip of an iceberg of staggering proportions. It is all the more puzzling to discover that a large proportion of these reports fall away at later stages in the criminal justice process. High attrition rates occur in other areas of crime too, such as robbery and burglary (Polk 1985), but often this is because the perpetrator of the crime is never caught. In sexual assault cases, it is more likely that there will be a suspect and yet attrition rates remain high. In Wright's study (see Chapter 1), of the 204 suspects arrested, only 35 (17 per cent) were found guilty of rape or attempted rape. In the remaining cases, either the prosecution did not proceed or the men were aquitted or found guilty of a lesser offence. Drawing on information supplied by 33 police forces in England and Wales, Lloyd and Walmsley estimated that in 1985 only 10 per cent of reported rapes and 50 per cent of rape prosecutions resulted in a conviction (Lloyd and Walmsley 1989). In the Home Office study conducted in the second half of 1985 (Grace *et al*. 1992), 25 per cent of the suspects were convicted of rape or attempted rape, a further 5 per cent were found guilty of lesser offences and the remaining 60 per cent were not convicted of any offence. In Scotland, Chambers and Millar found that 25 per cent of the reported rapes resulted in a conviction, but in more than a third of these the conviction was for a lesser or different offence (Chambers and Millar 1983).

Since the time periods covered by the research studies considered so far, another layer of decision-making has been introduced in England and Wales, with the creation of the CPS in 1985. The functions of investigation and prosecution have become separated, as has always been the case in Scotland, where prosecution is the responsibility of the Procurator Fiscal. Although the police still take the initial decision on whether or not to charge a suspect, the task of prosecution then passes to the independent prosecution service. At precisely the moment when the police in England and Wales were responding to criticisms and reviewing their policies in relation to crimes of violence against women, much of the initiative regarding the prosecution of offenders passed out of their control. In our own fieldwork, undertaken in the early 1990s, we were able to explore the impact of this development, both on decision-making processes within the police force and on attrition rates in relation to rape and sexual assault cases generally.

We identified four major points in the judicial process at which cases are excluded. The first occurs when a case is 'no-crimed' by the police, the second when the police fail to refer a case to the Crown Prosecution Service, the third when the CPS decides not to proceed or to reduce the charge to a less serious offence, and the last when the court dismisses the case or the jury finds the defendant 'not guilty'. We were interested in ascertaining which types of case were most likely to fall away and at which point in the process this attrition occurred.

## The practice of 'no criming'

In the first chapter, we presented the findings of earlier studies concerning the police practice of 'losing' cases that they regarded as hopeless and had no intention of investigating further, by adopting a strategy of 'no criming'. We saw that this was common practice in relation to crimes of rape and sexual assault and was of epidemic proportions in relation to domestic violence. Although it did occur in other categories of crime, the overall 'no-criming' rate had been estimated to be about 3 per cent (Bottomley and Coleman 1981). This indicates that crimes of violence against women were ranked extremely low in the list of police priorities and created the impression that thousands of women were making false allegations. In response to criticisms from women's groups and researchers, the guidelines for 'no criming' were tightened in a series of high level policy decisions. The Home Office led the way, by recommending that reports of serious sexual crimes should only be 'no crimed' if the complainant subsequently admitted that a false allegation had been made (Home Office circular 69/86).

These policy directives imposed from above were in direct conflict with the dictates of police culture, resonant with the assumption that complainants often make false allegations and waste police time. The tension between the new directives and the 'gut' feeling of police officers about these cases is evident from the findings of our research, both in some very revealing comments made by the officers we interviewed and in the data analysis.

During the interviews, several of the officers made reference to the 'bad old days' of harsh interrogation and unsympathetic handling of complainants, in the style so vividly depicted in the Thames Valley documentary (see Chapter 1). Since the furore generated by that episode, the police have operated under a clear instruction that no-one reporting a serious sexual assault is to be disbelieved. As an example of this new policy in action, one of the detective inspectors related a case in which a woman reported that she had been raped by a taxi driver but at the same time admitted that she might have dreamt it. The inspector acknowledged that in the past 'she would have been laughed out of the station', but in accordance with the new policies, the complaint was treated seriously. Semen found on her sheets matched with samples obtained from the taxi driver and he was convicted.

At one level, the officers seem committed to making the new policies work. The female officers who had been assigned to work with complainants under the new 'chaperone' system (discussed in detail in Chapter 6) were clearly attempting to provide a supportive service, despite the tendency for the rest of their work to 'pile up' while they did so and they were genuinely concerned that so few cases went to court. At another level, however, it is important to realize that old attitudes die hard and that conflicting pressures still exist. On the crucial question of false allegations for example, it was apparent that many officers still believed that these occur frequently. They gave hypothetical examples of mischievous reports of rape, such as the woman who has had a row with her boyfriend, the prostitute who has not been paid, the young woman who becomes pregnant or stays out all night and wishes to escape parental wrath. One inspector commented that the last three rapes he had dealt with were not rapes at all and another believed that 50 per cent of the rapes reported were probably false allegations.

There appears to be a singular lack of curiosity about why women should make false allegations. One officer asked to give a recent example of a false allegation, referred to a 15-year-old girl whom he could tell was 'sexually experienced' and whom he then recognized as having made a previous complaint. He seemed unsure as to whether or not the case had been referred to the child protection team. This is the kind of case which clearly merits further investigation. For a 15 year old to present herself at a police station in this way, she must be emotionally or mentally disturbed or genuinely in some danger; in either case, she requires help. The fact that she had made a previous complaint appeared to be viewed with some suspicion, although it could be precisely the experience of being sexually assaulted more than once which precipitated the complaint.

Notwithstanding the new sympathetic public face, the prevalence of such views regarding false allegations will inevitably influence the way that cases are processed. It helps to explain why the service has been slow to respond to the new policy guidelines on 'no criming', so that cases reported between September 1988 and September 1990 reveal a very similar pattern of 'no criming' to that found in studies undertaken earlier in the 1980s. Of the cases initially reported as rape, attempted rape or indecent assault during the two year period covered by the study, 38 per cent (116 out of 301) were 'no crimed'. When cases of rape and attempted rape were analyzed separately, the 'no criming' rate rose to 43 per cent (47 out of 109 cases). There were no significant changes during the two year research period, although there was a slight variation between the two police stations; at Holloway the 'no criming' rate was 47 per cent and at Kings Cross it was 42 per cent. This is higher than the rates reported in the two Home Office studies (Smith 1989a and Grace *et al.* 1992), although they relate to an earlier time period. It seems likely that our study provides a more complete picture, because of the exclusion from the other studies of cases crimed during the first month after reporting, as explained above.

Our findings indicate that despite the new guidelines on 'no criming', this category was still in frequent use at the end of the 1980s and in circumstances that fell well outside those officially sanctioned. In her Home Office study of two London boroughs, Smith (1989a) found that in 1984 the most usual explanation for 'no criming' was given as 'complaint withdrawn' and that it was a reduction in the use of this cate-gory that largely accounted for the drop in 'no criming' by 1986. Yet, as can be seen from Table 3.1, in more than half the 'no crimed' cases in our study, the justification still centred on the complainant's failure to substantiate the allegation. This includes complainants who have moved or disappeared, those who are reluctant to proceed for a variety of reasons and some who are seen as unreliable and prone to making false allegations or changing their story. The following examples serve to illustrate the diversity of situations covered by this category:

Victim adamant that no investigation take place, refused to substantiate.

Victim obtained an injunction against the suspect and withdrew allegation.

Victim, who was dumb, was transferred back to her own institution by the hospital without police being notified of address, but police were informed that victim is mentally ill and suffers delusions.

One case was still 'no crimed' under this heading, although the suspect admitted the offence and it was considered when he was charged with other similar offences. Another case was 'no crimed' because the complainant had a heart condition and could not cope with the ordeal of the court. Such complainant-initiated withdrawals were much more likely to occur in cases where there was some degree of prior acquaintance or intimacy between the complainant and the suspect. The greater the degree of intimacy, the more likely it is that the suspect will be able to exert pressure on the complainant for the case to be dropped. This raises the issue of whether or not the police should persist with an investigation after the woman has withdrawn her complaint, particularly where the case notes indicate the probability of undue pressure.

The other major justification for 'no criming' identified by Smith was 'insufficient evidence'. She found that by 1986 this category accounted for 61 per cent of the total 'no crimed' cases in her study. In our research, 'insufficient evidence to substantiate the allegation' provided the basis for 'no criming' in roughly one-third of the cases. The following examples are taken from this category:

> No physical evidence to substantiate allegation; victim was raped by boyfriend in 1986 and has had mental and emotional problems since; no forensic evidence, no corroboration, believed false allegation.

> Doctor's examination revealed injuries to be consistent with victim having fallen whilst inebriated; victim is alcoholic.

*Table 3.1* Reasons given for 'no criming', all cases

| Reason given | Number |
| --- | --- |
| Victim failed to substantiate allegation | 68 |
| Insufficient evidence to substantiate allegation | 33 |
| Child protection team dealing with the case | 5 |
| CPS advised no further action | 3 |
| Unable to identify suspect | 3 |
| Recording/administrative purposes only | 2 |
| No criminal action | 2 |
| Total cases 'no crimed' | 116 |

Such police-initiated withdrawals are based on police judgements as to the reliability of complainants as a source of evidence, including references to their mental stability. The need for corroboration indicates that the police were still failing to take cases seriously when they had doubts about the credibility of the witness, or believed that the case would not stand up in court.

It is likely that the rate of 'no criming' is even higher than that reflected in the record forms. One of the policewomen who collected some of the data for the project informed the researchers that two cases that had been 'no crimed' had been excluded from the data. In the first case, the complainant had come in to the police station claiming to have been raped but refusing to give details or to be medically examined and after two hours had left not to be seen again. In the second case, the complainant said she had been raped by her ex-boyfriend's friend, but had withdrawn the complaint the following day. If a case is 'no crimed' it does not mean that it cannot be re-categorized as a crime later. The same officer quoted a case that had originally been 'no crimed' but had been re-categorized as a crime when a number of similar offences were reported.

The five cases that were passed to the child protection team (see Table 3.1) were apparently 'no crimed' in order to prevent double counting. Since none of these cases went to court, it is reasonable to assume that the classification was not altered. The fact that some cases were 'no crimed' after the Crown Prosecution Service advised that no further action would be taken provides further evidence that 'no criming' decisions are still being made by the police at a late stage in the proceedings. For example in one case the police record reads: 'Victim and friends went to a party and got very drunk. She fell asleep and woke up when the suspect (a stranger) sat astride her. His erect penis was in his hand. He masturbated and then went off'. This was sent to the CPS who decided to take no further action. It was then reclassified by the police as 'no crime'.

There seems to be a confusion between criming and recording, so that it becomes possible for any case that does not proceed to fall under the 'no crime' category. The two cases that appear in Table 3.1 under the 'recording/administrative purposes only' category are very different from each other. In the first case, the home beat officer attended the suspect's home to speak informally about the incident reported, with no intention of pursuing the matter further. In the second case, by contrast, it was noted that the suspect was currently wanted by the police and once traced, could well be interviewed and possibly charged with the reported offence.

These categories are much wider than the recommendations of Home Office circular 69/86 that complaints of rape and sexual assault should not be 'no crimed' unless there is a retraction of the complaint and an admission of fabrication by the complainant. This failure to observe the official guidelines leads to an underestimation of the number of reported rapes and feeds the myth that false allegations are a common phenomenon. Women may decide for very good reasons that they do wish to proceed, perhaps because they have been threatened or because they feel unable to relive the assault and face a gruelling cross-examination in open court.

Whatever the reason for the reluctance, it is in the interests of the police to 'lose' such cases by 'no criming' them, in case they are otherwise considered to be not 'cleared up', which could reflect badly on police performance. In theory, this dilemma can be resolved, as Home Office regulations stipulate that cases can be deemed to be cleared up where they do not proceed to court, if the guilt of the accused is clear but the complainant refuses or is unable to give evidence, or the accused admits the offence but it is decided that no useful purpose would be served by proceeding with the charge. In practice, however, authority to clear up a serious sexual offence by means other than a prosecution lies with the divisional chief superintendent. As one detective inspector put it during an interview, this means that there is just as much paperwork involved in 'no criming' and then clearing up a rape or sexual assault as there is in proceeding with a charge. Several inspectors admitted that the temptation to 'no crime' cases still existed, because once something is crimed, there is no certainty that it will be possible to treat it as cleared up in the absence of a conviction. One inspector expressed his concern that an increase in sexual attacks recorded as crimes and then not cleared up would result in the fear of crime being greater than the real threat. This is a most revealing comment, as it ignores the evidence that many attacks are still unreported, while implying that many cases that are reported are not genuine.

In comparison with property crimes, there is a much greater likelihood that the victim of a sexual crime will be able to identify the perpetrator, particularly if he is not a total stranger, and consequently a higher arrest rate is to be expected. In 37 per cent (111 cases) an arrest was made. However, most of these cases fell by the wayside and did not proceed to a successful prosecution. In 22 of the cases in which arrests were made, the cases were subsequently 'no crimed', a reflection of the difficulty in proving beyond reasonable doubt that the crime took place, rather than the widespread existence of false allegations.

Once again, the category 'no crime' is very misleading in such cases, as well as flying in the face of circular 69/86.

In 1995, the Metropolitan Police issued yet another set of guidelines for investigators and chaperones in relation to the handling of serious sexual assaults (Metropolitan Police 1995). While broader than the Home Office guidelines, they are both comprehensive and precise, designed to produce greater rigour in dealing with such cases in the future. They stipulate that an allegation may be classified as 'no crime' only if: 'It is transferred to another division or there are substantial indications that the allegation is actually false' (ibid. 3). The following examples are then provided of the kinds of circumstances where it might be appropriate to 'no crime':

> When the victim admits the allegation is false and makes a statement to that effect; when medical or forensic evidence or that of an independent witness substantially contradicts, rather than does not support, the allegation; when there is substantial evidence that the victim is suffering from delusions or is making the allegation for some specific and inappropriate reason. Psychiatric impairment and alcohol or drug dependency are not the same as suffering from delusions, although there will be some cases where these conditions might contribute to an allegation being false.
>
> (Metropolitan Police 1995: 4)

Unless the police perception of the prevalence of false allegations is dramatically altered through training and experience, it seems likely that even these guidelines will prove to contain too many loopholes to address the problem of high rates of 'no criming'.

## The reclassification of offences

The persistence of the practice of 'no criming' is a major factor contributing to the high attrition rate in reported cases of rape and sexual assault. In addition, there is the process of reclassification, which in effect downgrades the crimes as initially reported and records them as less serious offences. If we turn to the 185 cases (out of the original 301) that were recorded as crimes, we find that 20 of these were reclassified by the police. Two of them were altered to indicate that a more serious offence had been committed, but the remaining 18 were downgraded. Two reports of rape and six reports of attempted rape were reclassified as indecent assault, one case of indecent assault was downgraded to indecent exposure and in the other nine cases the sexual aspect of the crime was removed altogether.

Clearly, it is in the interests of the complainant to reduce the charge if there is insufficient evidence to proceed with the more serious crime and such decisions have to be made on the basis of experience and judgement. However, for some of the cases in which the sexual classification was removed altogether, it appears that the police failed to recognize the importance of the sexual aspect of the crime. They include a case reclassified as robbery, although the suspect had allegedly squeezed the victim's breast and put his hand on her inner thigh, and a charge of grievous bodily harm (GBH) in which the attacker was described as ripping off the victim's shirt and bra and putting a finger in her vagina, slashing her breasts while threatening to cut them off. In another case reclassified as common assault, the victim regained consciousness to find the suspect urinating on her.

In one of the cases where we were able to interview the complainant (see Chapter 6), the woman, whom we refer to as Una, had reported her ex-husband as attempting to rape her. She had also been severely beaten up, but the charge was classified as indecent assault. Yet when this case came to court, even the indecent assault charge was unsuccessful and the defendant found not guilty. When interviewed, Una described what happened:

> I was married for seventeen years. I took a lot over the years for the sake of the children, but you get to the point when you think 'that's it'. You can't explain the kind of pressure I was under when I left, phone calls and hassle. I had an injunction as well to keep him away. But he just flipped. I thought he was going to kill me. I'd never seen him like that. He said 'Sleep with me and I'll give you some money'. Then he tried to rape me. I fought and he beat me up. My daughter was in the house and she heard everything. It took two calls to get the police and they took some time coming. When they saw how bad I looked they were sorry they had not been quicker. I was knocked about with bruises and cuts. The police arrested him for indecent assault. I said I wanted him arrested for attempted rape. He got off the indecent assault charge but was found guilty of ABH [actual bodily harm]. I would rather he had been found guilty of indecent assault.

In another case which had originally been classified as attempted rape, the suspect had stopped the victim in the street, forced her into a garden at knife-point, pushed her onto the ground, forcibly removed her knickers, masturbated over her and left. When the complainant had refused to proceed, the case had been reclassified as indecent assault. In quite a few of the cases in which the complainant was interviewed, the description of the attack seemed to merit a recording of attempted rape, as in Una's case, but the police had classified it as indecent assault. The distinction between the two remains unclear and there is no clear definition of intention to rape. Is verbal expression of intent sufficient or is genital contact required and if so, what kind of contact? Does throwing a woman on the ground, trying to remove her knickers and being fought off not constitute an intention to rape?

Indecent assault is defined as an assault which has some aspect of indecency about it, for example brushing against a body or breast grabbing. Sometimes the initial allegation may be changed after further questioning, so that an offence may initially be classed as attempted rape, but there may be insufficient evidence to prove that the suspect had intended to rape. During the interviews, police officers pointed out that a lesser charge was often more likely to secure a conviction. It also follows that if the crime is not cleared up, it looks better in the statistics if it is a less serious crime. One senior policewoman helped to throw some light on possible reasons for downgrading serious crimes in this way. She recounted how, on returning to the station from other duties at the end of 1988, she had taken a statement from a rape victim who did not wish to proceed with the case. In accordance with previous practice, she had 'no crimed' the report and was reprimanded for doing so. She was informed that the new guidelines related to rape reports only and was asked if the report could be reclassified as indecent assault, in which case it could then be 'no crimed'. Here is a vivid illustration of the dilemma faced by the police as they attempt to reconcile the requirement to treat reports of rape seriously and the requirement to produce statistics which present their own performance as crime controllers in a favourable light.

## 'Crimed' cases not referred to the CPS

By no means were all the 185 cases 'crimed' by the police forwarded to the Crown Prosecution Service. In 88 cases of assaults by strangers, the attacker was never identified, in 4 cases the suspect was issued with an official caution and in 10 the police decided to take no further action. This decision was usually based on the unavailability of the complainant or her unwillingness to pursue the complaint. For example, in one case involving indecent assault by an employer, the case note reads: 'Victim unwilling to attend court. Suspect questioned, kept on file'. In a case of rape in which the police took no further action, the complainant withdrew her statement and removed the forensic evidence. In all, 88 cases were forwarded to the CPS, less than a third of the original 301 reported to the police. They included five cases subsequently 'no crimed' by the police, suggesting that the classification process takes place over a considerable period of time.

In their study of how police officers and prosecutors make decisions in relation to criminal cases, McConville *et al.* (1991) conclude that the impact of law reform is invariably neutralized by the operation of police culture and that new rules are circumvented, enabling the 'crime control' philosophy of the police to survive any attempts at imposing due process principles upon them.[2] The McConville study covered a wide spectrum of cases drawn from three police stations and only included six cases of rape and sexual assault. Our study by contrast focuses specifically on this type of crime, examining the evolving relationship between the police and the CPS in the light of the radical policy shifts that have occurred in recent years. While not underestimating the effects of the 'crime control' imperative, we believe that a much more complex dynamic is at work.

The Metropolitan Police Force is about halfway down a league table of cautioning rates and is under pressure to caution offenders more frequently, rather than to put 'cases that won't go anywhere' through to the CPS. As one of the detective inspectors we interviewed explained:

> The CPS won't take cases that the police would have taken pre-1985, but if the police were still responsible for prosecutions now, they would probably be subject to same pressures as the CPS is experiencing. There are greater pressures to caution nowadays, for example first time shoplifters, but not in cases of rape. There are cases where the police would want to 'give it a run', particularly if the victim is strong, but the CPS is often reluctant. As an example, there was a case where a baby was shaken so hard that its brain was damaged and almost certainly one of the parents was responsible, but the baby couldn't give evidence and it wasn't possible to pin it down to one or the other of the parents, so the CPS wouldn't proceed.

A senior officer recounted a case of indecency to children in which the police worked hard identifying suspects, and interviewing children and adults, but when the case went to court, the CPS decided to offer no evidence. The police were then involved in a considerable amount of painstaking work to fulfil all the criteria that the Director of Public Prosecutions demanded before the case could be reinstated. From the police officer's perspective, this felt like discouragement, although he knew that the CPS would say that the police had not prepared the case properly.

One relatively experienced female officer said that she had dealt with ten sexual assault cases, none of which went to court. Some were dropped because the victim did not wish to proceed, in one the offender was not caught, and in the rest the CPS took no further action. The officer commented that she had become too involved in the cases to take an objective view of the CPS decisions, but admitted that it is always hard to explain to a woman why her case does not proceed. She also acknowledged that there were a large number of acquittals, particularly in cases of non-stranger rape 'as it is a case of his word against hers'. She then made a particularly revealing comment:

> The CPS is open to persuasion and will sometimes go ahead with a case they would prefer to drop. They would do their best in such cases but they are not always on top of the job, although they are improving. They get paid much less than the defence lawyers and (unlike them) the success of their career doesn't depend on their success rate.

As the police are constantly placed in the position of having to 'second guess' what the Crown Prosecution Service will do, their beliefs about the criteria used by the Service will have a crucial influence on their decisions concerning which cases to send forward to the CPS and which cases are 'no-hopers'. One of the chief superintendents commented: 'Unfortunately, a number of victims are not regarded by the CPS as competent witnesses because of emotional or other difficulties, so these cases don't go to court'. A woman officer believed that

> Rapes of prostitutes are difficult to get to court because the CPS isn't prepared to go ahead. Stranger rapes are the easiest to get through the initial stages as far as the CPS and then to secure a conviction if there is evidence.

In our study, two cases involving complainants identified as prostitutes did proceed to court but in neither case was the suspect charged with rape. The first case was reported as attempted rape but subsequently downgraded to indecent assault. The woman had agreed to have sex for a fixed sum but the man had refused to pay and had pulled her underwear down in the street. The police had actually observed the offence occurring and so could provide the necessary corroboration. In the second case the suspect picked up the prostitute and took her to his home. There he bound and gagged her, beat her and threatened to kill her. He raped and buggered her. At court, the defendant was sentenced to five years for threat to kill, seven years for indecent assault, five years for assault with intent to commit buggery and five years for actual bodily harm (ABH). The rape charge was dropped.

The police have been pressed hard to improve the standard of victim care, thereby encouraging more women who have been sexually assaulted by men they know to come forward. At the same time, they are under considerable political pressure to improve clear up rates while relinquishing control of the prosecution role to the CPS. In responding to these contradictory expectations, it is the pressure coming from the politicians, the CPS and the courts that carries the greatest weight, and the combined effect of these pressures seems likely to increase the attrition rates rather than reduce them. As one chief superintendent put it: 'In the old days, the police had a duty to "give it a run" whenever the law had been broken, but now they almost have a duty to discontinue'. However, the police are not always successful in anticipating what action the CPS will take. Despite their apparently stringent screening procedures, passing through the CPS gateway provided absolutely no guarantee that a successful prosecution would ensue and the processes of attrition continued unabated.

## The crown prosecution service and the courts

In approximately one-fifth of the cases referred to the Crown Prosecution Service (17 out of 88), the CPS decided to take no further action. Of the 71 cases that did proceed, 41 resulted in a conviction (although one of these was quashed on appeal) and in a further three, the offender was detained under the Mental Health Act. The remaining 27 cases fell away at various stages of the proceedings; in two cases the suspect failed to appear in court; in a number of others the proceedings were discontinued and the rest culminated in a finding of not guilty. It is worth noting that the figure of 40 convictions (excluding the one quashed on appeal) provides a false picture of the number of offenders convicted, as in some cases suspects were sentenced for a number of offences simultaneously. In the Holloway data for example, it is made clear that a sentence of one month's imprisonment for indecent assault indicated against seven cases was in fact the same offender being convicted on one occasion for all seven crimes.

In the Islington data the picture is less clear. The information 'three year's youth custody for indecent assault concurrent with five other counts' appears against five different cases but differences in the age and race classification of suspects point to the probability that two, or perhaps three, offenders were involved in these cases. An alternative explanation is that the police were over-zealous in attempting to improve their clear up figures, by persuading offenders to ask for other offences to be taken into consideration. This explanation is given plausibility by the following account from a victim of one of these five attacks:

> They took a statement. The police said it had happened to two other women the same night and they had said he was white. I had said he was definitely dark skinned. Some months later I bought a local paper and in it there was this article saying a man had been arrested for offences in the area. He sort of fitted the description. So I rang the detective again and he said 'Yes, it's the same person and he's been arrested and prosecuted'. I think it was in May there was another article saying that he'd been charged with four offences. Then I was looking through the cuttings again and it only just dawned on me that I don't think he was charged with what he did to me, because the dates in the paper were different, they were after it happened to me. I mean, it could have been someone else.

Even allowing for a certain amount of double-counting, a success rate of 43 (including the three detained under the Mental Health Act) out of 71 might seem reasonable taken in isolation. However, for an accurate assessment of 'success' to be made, these figures have to seen in the context of the high rates of attrition which have already occurred at earlier stages in the reporting process, and the fact that the convictions were often for a lesser charge.

Our interview with the branch crown prosecutor helped to throw some light on the observations made by the police officers we had interviewed. The prosecutor informed us that although the CPS does collect statistics, there is no breakdown which indicates the rate of attrition of individual categories of crime and that monitoring is done by ensuring that quality standards are maintained, rather than through the collection of statistics. There is a scrutiny of individual cases to see why they were lost, focusing particularly on the jury verdict and the direction given to the jury by the judge. He stated that if many cases were being lost in court, the CPS lawyers would have to take this into account in deciding whether or not to prosecute, but he also insisted that the CPS aims to achieve uniformity and consistency; it is a national service with a code of practice that sets down the criteria to be used when initiating criminal proceedings.

The account which follows draws both from the comments made by the prosecutor during the interview and from the *Code for Crown Prosecutors* (CPS 1992) in use at the time of the interview. There are two main criteria which are used to determine whether or not to proceed with a particular case: the first relates to the sufficiency of the evidence and the second to whether or not prosecution is in the public interest. In relation to the first, the prosecutor is required to consider a number of questions:

> Does it appear that a witness is exaggerating or that his [sic] memory is faulty, or that he is either hostile or friendly to the accused, or may otherwise be unreliable?

> Has a witness a motive for telling less than the whole truth?

> Are there matters which might properly be put to a witness by the defence to attack his credibility?

> What sort of impression is the witness likely to make? How is he likely to stand up to cross-examination?

> Does he suffer from any physical or mental disability which is likely to affect his credibility?

These questions are undoubtedly relevant from the point of view of a prosecutor considering whether a defence lawyer might make mincemeat of a key prosecution witness; they also confirm the police view of the type of cases most likely to secure a conviction, the prototype of which is the rape of a 'respectable' woman by a stranger.

Although the public interest criteria require the prosecutor to weigh the likely penalty with the likely length and cost of the proceedings, the branch prosecutor insisted that at the more serious end of the spectrum, there should be no equivocation: sexual assaults on children should always be regarded seriously, as should offences against adults, such as rape, which amount to gross personal violation. In such cases, where the crown prosecutor is satisfied as to the sufficiency of the evidence, there will seldom be any doubt that prosecution will be in the public interest. On the other hand, he admitted that the complainant's attitude may be a decisive factor. In some cases, it will be appropriate to take account of the attitude of the complainant who notified the police but later expressed a wish that no action be taken. It may be that in these circumstances proceedings should not be pursued unless there is suspicion that the change of heart was activated by fear or the offence was of some gravity.

The code confirms that the police are very much the junior partner when it comes to decisions concerning prosecution:

> Unless, of course, advice has been given at a preliminary stage, the police decision to institute proceedings should never be met with passive acquiescence but must always be the subject of review....It will be the normal practice to consult the police whenever it is proposed to discontinue proceedings instituted by them. The level of consultation will depend on the particular circumstances of the case or the accused, but the final decision will rest with the Crown Prosecutor.
>
> (CPS 1992)

The branch prosecutor confirmed that the CPS carefully guards its independence, which is enshrined in statute. He said that the service finds itself in some difficulty where it is involved in working parties or in committees where individual cases are raised. It wishes to be informed, but does not want to be subjected to particular sectional pressures and interests. The CPS has an observer role at Victim Support meetings but needs to preserve its independence, as public interest takes priority over the interests of the victim where these conflict.

Although the prosecutor insisted that victim care was of major concern to the CPS, it was difficult to see how this could be given practical effect. He acknowledged a certain lack of symmetry in the trial situation, in so far as the defence lawyer's prime duty is to the defence, whereas the prosecution is there to present evidence on behalf of the court in the interests of justice, and so is not there in a strictly adversarial role. However, he did not consider the idea of the woman having her own lawyer fitted well with our system of justice and viewed it as unnecessary, in view of the prosecution concern with the administration of evidence and the rules of law concerning what is admissible. He confirmed that it was against the ethics of the bar to prepare a witness for the trial. A barrister might introduce him- or herself to the complainant but would not discuss the details of the case. Whatever the arguments in favour of such an ethic, it effectively rules out any role for the prosecuting counsel in helping to make the courtroom a less hostile environment for complainants.

In the revised version of the Code published in 1994, a number of changes were introduced, including the addition of some anti-discrimination guidelines: 'Crown Prosecutors must be fair, independent and objective. They must not let their personal views of ethnic or national origin, sex, religious beliefs, political views or sexual prefer-ence of the offender, victim or witness influence their decisions' (CPS 1994a: 3).

Women's organizations interested in monitoring the work of the CPS in relation to rape prosecutions claim that there is 'no evidence that the new Code has resulted in fairer judgment' (Women Against Rape and Legal Action for Women 1995: 6). They point out that women who have a history of mental illness or who have learning disabilities are regarded as incapable of understanding what was happening to them and therefore of withholding their consent to sex; so their cases are dropped on the basis of lack of evidence. The irony is that the CPS lawyer makes these judgements without ever meeting the witnesses. It also seems to contradict the CPS claim to be concerned with witness care.

It was the Royal Commission on Criminal Justice reporting in 1981 that recommended the setting up of an independent prosecution service with the intention of raising standards in this area of criminal justice. A Metropolitan Police commander confided to David Rose, 'There were times when we used to prosecute on the basis of a case scrawled on the back of a fag packet' (Rose 1996b: 2). Rose believes that without the creation of the CPS, many people would have been wrongly prosecuted and perhaps wrongly convicted over the period of its existence. Nevertheless, the Service has been subjected to a number of criticisms from various quarters and these are no longer confined to comments on its early teething problems, attributable to understaffing and the speed with which it was set up. The criticisms fall into three main categories: first, the way in which the CPS makes prosecution decisions, second, the way in which cases are handled once a prosecu-tion decision has been made and third, the way in which the organization is structured and managed and its lack of accountability.

## Deciding whether to prosecute

The criticisms are by no means confined to CPS decision-making in relation to sexual offences. The number of cases which are dropped after a hearing at the magistrates' court has been increasing steadily; reasons for non-continuation include insufficient evidence, the disappearance of witnesses or because the CPS decided it was 'not in the public interest' to prosecute. Complainants and their relatives who feel particularly aggrieved when this happens and who are able and prepared to spend their own money to pursue the matter further, have the option of a private prosecution, although the Director of Public Prosecutions still has the power to prevent the case proceeding on the grounds that it is not in the public interest.

In 1986, the parents of a man murdered by a drug pusher brought the first successful private prosecution for manslaughter and since then such prosecutions have become increasingly common. Sometimes, embarking on a private prosecution has the effect of making the CPS change its mind and it takes over the prosecution. The original plaintiffs then lose control of the proceedings and will be powerless to intervene if the charge is downgraded to a lesser offence, but at least the case does go forward. If they go it alone while the CPS remains aloof, they face almost insurmountable obstacles in obtaining the necessary evidence as the witness statements, police reports and forensic analyses relating to the case remain confidential (*Independent on Sunday*, 30 April 1995). David Rose gives an account of the case of Christopher Davis, accused of raping two prostitutes at knife point. Although the two women told almost identical stories and Davis already had a conviction for abduction and assault, the CPS considered that a jury might not accept the evidence of prostitutes and decided not to proceed. The women battled for three and a half years to bring the first private prosecution for rape. The jury was unanimous in finding him guilty and he was sentenced to eleven years. An independent barrister had advised the CPS that it ought to prosecute in this particular case on public interest grounds as Davis was 'a very dangerous man who would have gone on to rape again' (Rose 1996b: 2).

The failure of the Crown Prosecution Service to prosecute in such cases means that the women involved are denied public recognition for the injury they have suffered as well as being deprived of access to justice. A number of feminist pressure groups, including Women Against Rape (WAR) and Legal Action for Women (LAW), combined to produce a dossier of fifteen cases in which the CPS decided not to prosecute. Women Against Rape and Legal Action for Women felt so strongly about these particular cases that they wrote to the Director of Public Prosecutions on behalf of the women asking for a review of the decisions, with little success. They make the following points:

> When 11 out of 12 rape survivors do not report to the police, the one woman who does report, and who is ready to put herself through a trial, is invaluable in identifying, condemning and isolating rapists – yet the service her action can be to society generally is regularly disregarded by CPS lawyers. The survivor who is turned down by the CPS loses not only the freedom from fear she would gain if the man were imprisoned, but public recognition of the harm she has suffered and State condemnation of her attacker, which reasserts her own social worth and her social power against the man who raped her. This is a vital part of her recovery....Those who have been convicted of a crime they didn't commit are not the only victims of a 'miscarriage of justice'; so are those who have suffered a crime and are denied justice: public acknowledgement of what they have undergone and public condemnation of their assailant.
>
> (WAR/LAW 1995: 1 and 9)

Women Against Rape and Legal Action for Women point out that the most striking feature of the cases in their dossier is that either the victims had low social status or social power and/or their attackers had high social status or power. Five of the victims were children, three were women with disabilities, three were black, one an immigrant and two were students. Seven were raped at home, one in a hospital, one by a policeman and four by acquaintances (WAR/LAW 1995). It is clear that there is a 'hierarchy of credibility' (Becker 1967) at work here, so that witnesses who are less articulate, less fluent in English and unlikely to make 'good witnesses' are systematically denied justice.

Rose cites the example of a working class Irish girl whose case was dropped by the CPS despite her extensive injuries, on the grounds that she had had a previous sexual relationship with her attacker, that they had both drunk alcohol and that she had fainted during the attack and so was unsure as to whether or not intercourse had taken place. The CPS discontinued the case without waiting for vital forensic evidence, involving the analysis of blood stains on a knife owned by the suspect and identified by the victim as the weapon used in the attack. (Rose 1996a: 139)

The 'miscarriages of justice' reported by Women Against Rape and

by Rose stand in sharp contrast to the decision of the CPS to prosecute in the case of Austen Donnellan. In this case, there had been no
previous sexual relationship between the two students, but they had
been seen kissing at a Christmas party, both were very drunk and the
complainant could not remember exactly what happened as she had
passed out (Lees 1997a: 81). The woman in this case had not asked for
a prosecution and had only reported the rape to the college authorities
because she had to attend lectures with Donnellan after the alleged
rape. It was Donnellan who then reported the accusation to the police.
The prosecution can therefore only be seen as 'in the public interest' in
the sense that it allowed Donnellan to clear his name. As the authors
of the WAR dossier point out, the case had the effect of discrediting
rape trials as unfair to men while discouraging women from reporting
and pursuing cases. It is difficult to believe that the CPS could not have
anticipated such an outcome.

In 1994 the CPS discontinued 160,000 criminal prosecutions, which
represented 11 per cent of the total number of recorded crimes and an
increase of about 50 per cent in comparison to its first year of operation (CPS 1995). Despite this draconian 'weeding out' of cases, a
research study undertaken for the Royal Commission on Criminal
Justice found that more than half the acquittals in 1993 were either
ordered by the judge before the trial began or directed by the judge at
the close of the trial. The researchers estimate that the majority of
those acquittals were foreseeable, due to the weakness of the evidence
and they regard these findings as an indictment of the CPS (Block *et
al.* 1993). Rose endorses this view and offers the following comment:

> The CPS seems to be operating in an almost haphazard fashion:
> throwing out cases with utmost expedition where conviction might
> have been possible, while pressing ahead with others where it
> seems most improbable.
>
> (Rose 1996a: 143)

It seems that there is considerable variation between different branches
of the CPS, despite the existence of the Code for Crown Prosecutors.

### The process of prosecution

The second major criticism of the CPS concerns the way in which it
handles cases once it has decided to proceed with a prosecution.
Members of Women Against Rape describe how they have had to
watch helplessly while prosecutions failed because crucial facts were

not emphasized or not even raised by the prosecution barrister. In one particular case, the prosecution asked the complainant a series of irrelevant intimate details about the rape while failing to ask her crucial questions concerning the accused's violent treatment of her. When she turned to WAR for help and a WAR representative attempted to intervene, the representative was accused of 'coaching' the witness. The trial was delayed while the matter was investigated and although the representative was exonerated, the misrepresentation of evidence was not corrected and the jury acquitted the suspect.

It is clearly wrong that the rule against 'coaching' witnesses should apply to a women's organization offering support and advice to women complainants, who are not even entitled to their own legal representation in court. Complainants invariably need protection from the harsh interrogation which is the hallmark of defence lawyers, making full use of the adversarial system to obtain the best possible outcome for their clients. All too often, complainants also need protection from the prosecution barrister; obsessed by the 'no coaching' rule, he or she remains aloof, meeting the complainant only briefly or not at all. This contrasts sharply with the close working relationship which often develops between defendants and defence barristers and adds to the complainant's sense of isolation and betrayal. As one of the interviewees in a study of rape complainants undertaken by Victim Support expressed it:

> I would have liked to have met the CPS before the case. I was on his side but there was no chance to get a rapport. You are anxious anyway and it makes it worse that you don't know who is who.
>
> (Victim Support 1996: 25)

The woman interviewed goes on to explain that in this particular case a retrial was ordered at a very late stage in the proceedings. There was no explanation for this, but the complainant was instructed not to mention the first trial or the case would be thrown out. This proved extremely difficult, as the defence lawyer seemed determined to trick her into making a reference to the first trial. She felt 'totally and utterly unsupported' by the CPS lawyer, who remained silent. 'There seemed to be a hidden agenda. I was a pawn in their game. It was a historical and political battle between the egos of the two barristers and I was the victim' (Victim Support 1996: 26).

CPS lawyers in England and Wales are not permitted to meet with witnesses before a trial, except to introduce themselves. This is not the case in Scotland. Indeed, as Liz Kelly *et al.* (1998) point out, 'Most other common law legal systems now view contact between victim/witnesses as vital components of case preparation'. For example, in Northern Ireland the victim is in a position to gain first hand information from the prosecution prior to the decision to prosecute. In cases where witness credibility is important, the Northern Ireland CPS regards it as essential that a meeting with the witness takes place both before the decision to prosecute and, if the case goes to trial, after the court hearing. The prosecution also meets with the witness to go through her statement. The guidelines for prosecutors specify that the consultation should take place with a police officer present; it is the officer's responsibility to accompany the witness to the interview. As a result of these procedures, the proportion of cases resulting in directed acquittals is substantially lower in Northern Ireland than in England and Wales.

The CPS in England and Wales is not totally unresponsive on this issue. In December 1997 the CPS website included the following:

> The CPS is fully committed to taking all practicable steps to help victims through the often difficult experience of becoming involved in the criminal justice system. The recently revised Victim's Charter sets out the service which victims can expect from the CPS, police, courts, witness service and others. These commitments will help to ensure that victims are better informed both about their own case and the way in which the criminal justice system works. The Charter also tells victims how to proceed if they are not satisfied with any aspect of the way in which the CPS or any of the other agencies has dealt with their case. The CPS is continuing to work with the police, the courts and the probation service to identify other ways to help victims. Discussions are underway to help assess the impact of a crime on the victim so their view can be taken into account whenever appropriate. A pilot scheme to develop this will start during 1996–7.
>
> (CPS website, December 1997)

It is to be hoped that some radical changes will be implemented as a consequence of all these initiatives, rather than a few cosmetic changes, as current research evidence points to widespread and deep-seated dissatisfaction, due largely to a failure of communication. In those cases in which the charge is downgraded to a less serious offence in an attempt to persuade the suspect to plead guilty, the sense of betrayal is compounded. The Victim Support study included a questionnaire survey on the treatment of rape complainants. This revealed that where charges were downgraded, fewer than one-third of the women were informed of the CPS reasons. In some cases, complainants said that they felt under pressure to agree to a downgrading. Two of the eleven women interviewed reported being asked by the CPS on the day of the trial whether they would accept a guilty plea to a charge of indecent assault:

> Both of these women were asked to make this decision in a very short space of time, just before they were due to give evidence, without any proper support or advice. They were persuaded that by accepting the plea they would be saved from the trauma of giving evidence, as well as allowing them to leave the court building before the defendant and his supporters came out. They believed that the defendant would still receive a custodial sentence. The outcome in each instance was that the defendant only received a fine. They both feel that they made their decision based on inaccurate reassurances from the CPS.
>
> (Victim Support 1996: 55)

There are a number of pressures which encourage defendants to plead guilty to a lesser offence, not least the prospect of a more lenient sentence than they would receive if they were to be convicted after pleading not guilty. If they plead guilty to an offence which can be dealt with summarily in the magistrates' court, the case will be heard and a decision reached much more quickly than if the case were to proceed to a full trial. From the point of view of the CPS, this is a desirable outcome, saving both time and money. If it is not possible to prevent a case proceeding to the Crown Court, the CPS still considers it worthwhile to avoid a full trial through the process of accepting guilty pleas (CPS 1994a: section 9). The result is a large number of 'cracked trials', i.e. cases where defendants elect jury trial but then change their plea to guilty on the morning of the case, as a result of the inducements offered to them by defence counsel at the eleventh hour (Rose 1996a: 152). Despite CPS protestations to the contrary, this process of charge reduction often leads to inappropriately lenient penalties. It is driven by the need to save money rather than the requirements of justice. As one solicitor put it:

> The CPS wins because it has a victory. The courts win because they see their backlog of cases reduced. The defendant wins because he gets a fine instead of a prison sentence. The Treasury

wins because the cheap option has been followed. Everyone wins except the victim.

(*Independent on Sunday*, 30 April 1995)

This may be oversimplified, as the outcome is certainly not in the interests of the defendant if he (or she) is innocent and has been denied a proper trial; also, it could be of considerable benefit to the victim to have the matter dealt with speedily and to avoid the trauma of having to appear on the witness stand.

Research by Cretney and Davis (1997) found that charge reduction was particularly common in cases of domestic violence, where reducing charges of actual bodily harm to common assault was almost routine, enabling such cases to be dealt with by magistrates. In their study of 448 assault cases prosecuted in the Bristol courts between January and October 1993, Cretney and Davis found that 94 per cent of domestic cases , compared with 79 per cent of non-domestic cases, were disposed of in this way. From a lawyer's perspective, this was seen to have three clear advantages: speed of processing, greater certainty of outcome and cost reduction. The CPS lawyers interviewed by Cretney and Davis did not believe that these considerations militated against the interests of complainants. They argued that speed reduces the period of uncertainty while making the most of the complainant's original commitment to prosecution. They also claim that judges dislike 'domestic' cases and are more likely than magistrates to impose inadequate sentences and even to reprimand prosecutors for proceeding with such cases (Cretney and Davis 1997: 149). The complainants interviewed by Cretney and Davis took a different view, believing that downgrading the charge trivialized their experience of injury and suffering, often endured over a long period of time. Reducing the charge had implications for the way the evidence was presented, so that some of the women reported that prosecutors had downplayed the degree of the violence involved, in order to make it fit more easily with the revised charge. In one case

the prosecutor, having accepted a defence plea to common assault (the original charge was ABH) had to pick his way through the original police summary of the incident: 'kicking and punching' became 'slapping'; threats with a knife became the act of 'showing' the victim a knife. On conclusion of the case the prosecutor's comment to us was: 'It's not exactly what happened but it's better than nothing'.

(Cretney and Davis 1997: 151)

When Kelly *et al.* (1998) tracked 34 defendants who had been charged in connection with offences of domestic violence, they found that 8 charges had been reduced by the CPS, including 40 per cent of ABH charges being reduced to common assault. They also reported an expectation on the part of the CPS that women will withdraw, so that they constantly ask the police to confirm that the victim wishes to proceed. This expectation is communicated to police officers with the danger that they may then be less supportive of the woman; this in turn may feed into her ambivalence about prosecution, rather than strengthening her resolve to press charges.

In a letter to *The Times* (15 September 1995), Barbara Mills, the Director of Public Prosecutions, rejected criticisms that the CPS was dominated by a culture of 'excessive caution' or by budgetary constraints in making prosecution decisions. She insisted that every case had to meet the test of whether or not there was sufficient evidence to make a conviction more likely than not. She commented: 'Although we discontinue only 11.7 per cent of cases, it does not follow that victims find it easy to accept that the case does not meet the tests' and she added that if the evidence was not there, it was their duty not to proceed. Under the CPS *Code for Crown Prosecutors*, any case meeting the two tests of sufficiency of evidence and whether prosecution was in the public interest would be prosecuted and she believed that 'by far the bulk of cases' meeting these tests were prosecuted.

It is not surprising that many cases which would easily satisfy the requirement applied by magistrates at committal, that there is a case to answer, fail to pass the much more stringent tests laid down in the Code. There is also a degree of tension between the two tests enshrined in the Code. For example, the list of public interest factors in favour of prosecution include the following:

> The more serious the offence, the more likely it is that a prosecution will be needed; A prosecution is likely to be needed if the victim of the offence was vulnerable, has been put in considerable fear or suffered personal attack, damage or disturbance; If a weapon was used or violence was threatened during the commission of the offence.
>
> (CPS 1994a: section 6.4)

Yet it is precisely the most vulnerable victims whose cases may be dropped for evidential reasons:

Is it likely that a confession is unreliable, for example, because of the defendant's age, intelligence or lack of understanding?

Is the witness's background likely to weaken the prosecution case? For example, does the witness have any dubious motive that may affect his or her attitude to the case...?

(CPS 1994a: section 5.3)

It is difficult to see how the CPS can do other than drop cases when they are required to proceed only with those that have a reasonable chance of resulting in a conviction. Despite Barbara Mills' insistence that 'Conviction rates play no part whatever' (*The Times*, 15 September 1995), it is likely that the CPS is subjected to pressures from above. A detective inspector told us in December 1994 that a CPS branch prosecutor friend of his had been rapped across the knuckles for committing too many cases to the Crown Court which resulted in acquittals. This would be likely to affect his promotion prospects if it continued. A similar explanation is given for why so many cases in the United States are dropped. According to Frohmann (1991), the promotion policy of the District Attorney's office encourages prosecutors to accept only 'strong' or 'winnable' cases for prosecution by using conviction rates as a measure of prosecutorial performance. Taking risks is discouraged as 'not guilty' verdicts are used as an indicator of prosecutorial incompetence. Prosecutors are given credit for the number of cases they reject in recognition of their commitment to the organizational concern of reducing the case load and saving money.

## CPS management and accountability

This brings us to the third major criticism of the CPS, concerning the way in which it is managed and held to account for its decisions. Since 1992 CPS staff have been required to meet 'performance indicator' targets, designed to ensure that cases which are to be dropped are thrown out as early as possible. In response to the demands of the Treasury and its own senior managers, the Service has suffered cutbacks in resources and personnel available for casework, while witnessing an expanding headquarters bureaucracy at the top. A Mori survey of lawyers, commissioned by their union, the First Division Association, found that more than a third of the staff expressed their deep concern about the direction of the organization and its ability to perform its public role (*Guardian*, 19 November 1996: 2). Neil Addison, a senior crown prosecutor for eight years, explains:

What has gone wrong is not the fault of the ordinary staff. They are merely the infantry trying to do their best. The fault lies in the overcentralized bureaucratic, autocratic management structure and the lack of any clear idea of what the CPS exists to achieve.

(*Guardian*, 30 November 1996)

This development was quite contrary to the vision of the Royal Commission on Criminal Justice that in 1981 recommended the setting up of the CPS; it had visualized a locally-based, decentralized prosecution service with a local chief crown prosecutor co-equal with the chief constable and responsible for prosecutions within the same area.

During its first decade of existence, control from the centre has intensified and in the latest restructuring thirteen chief prosecutors became responsible for large areas of the country, not related in any way to police force areas, Crown Court circuits or regional crime squad boundaries. According to Addison, this was a deliberate ploy to break the influence of local management and make everyone responsive to the cult of 'corporate loyalty': 'There is no realisation that the ultimate role of a prosecuting organization is law enforcement and that prosecuting decisions are not simply legal but have implications for policing and law and order generally' (*Guardian*, 30 November 1996).

The contrast between the anxieties expressed by the rank and file members of staff and the complacency of those at the top could not be greater. It is epitomized in the 1994 report of the head of the CPS, Director of Public Prosecutions Barbara Mills. She boasts of providing the public with a high quality and efficient public prosecution service. The doubling of the number of cases discontinued since the late 1980s is laid firmly at the door of the police for not making sufficient evidence available to provide a realistic prospect of conviction (CPS 1994b).

Relationships between the police and the CPS have reached an all time low and it is difficult to see how they can be improved while the CPS remains arrogant and aloof, deliberately creating structures which set it apart from the rest of the criminal justice system. The exasperation felt by senior police officers is well-expressed by chief constable Charles Pollard of the Thames Valley Police:

As a chief constable, I have to make decisions which are subject to scrutiny. But the CPS can act with effective autonomy, despite its enormous authority in deciding who should be prosecuted and who should not. It claims to act in the public interest, but it has absolutely no contact with the public. There needs to be a means of creating a dialogue to make the CPS accountable. Meanwhile, when the CPS makes decisions which force us to discontinue, it is us, the police, who have to tell the victim.

(Rose 1996a: 143–4)

In response to the growing criticisms of the CPS from the police and from organizations concerned with the welfare of victims, the previous government considered changes among which were: basing some CPS lawyers at major police stations; relaxing the '51 per cent chance of conviction' rule and giving the police a mechanism by which they could challenge CPS decisions not to pursue prosecutions (*Independent*, 5 December 1995). According to Neil Addison:

The CPS monolith should be broken up, with local chief prosecutors appointed for each police force area. These posts should be publicly advertised and not mere internal appointments. There should also be an independent board of inspectors comprising judges, magistrates, police and lawyers to inspect and report on prosecution standards.

(*Guardian*, 30 November 1996)

There has been a partial response to these criticisms. In an Explanatory Memorandum for use in connection with the *Code for Crown Prosecutors*, the '51 per cent rule' is rejected because it might 'convey the impression that the decision-making process is susceptible of very precise numerical definition', but the 'realistic prospect of conviction' test remains, defined as a case in which 'a jury or bench of magistrates, properly directed in accordance with the law, is more likely than not to convict the defendant of the charge alleged' (CPS 1996: 6). Pilot schemes were established in January 1996 in eleven police force areas for lawyers to work in police stations and administrative support units and the CPS and police forces are working together on 'the largest ever joint training scheme' (CPS Website November 1997). Also in January 1996, a CPS Inspectorate was established to ensure the maintenance and improvement of quality decision-making within the CPS.

In January 1998, the Inspectorate published its first study of how the CPS deals with a particular type of case; child abuse provided the focus for the study. Dramatic differences were found in conviction rates across the six area branches selected, ranging from 38 per cent to 80 per cent. Despite CPS policy that the best interests of the child are paramount when decisions are made concerning the need for therapy, some crown prosecutors were not aware of the policy and believed that therapy should be discouraged or prohibited while criminal proceedings were continuing. The report commented on the lack of communication between the CPS and the police, so that important information was often missing. Barristers were also frequently not supplied with full background information nor even told how a child wanted to give evidence; consequently children were not being offered the choice of videotape, video link or screens, nor the possibility of a familiarization visit to the courtroom before the trial (CPS Inspectorate 1998). It is to be hoped that the Service will respond to criticisms emanating from its own inspectorate and become less complacent and less secretive, recognizing the need for greater public accountability for its decisions and for greater co-operation with other parts of the criminal justice system.

## The Glidewell report: review of the CPS

As a consequence of the growing chorus of criticisms of the CPS, the Labour government, which came to power in May 1997, took immediate action on this issue. First, the trend towards over-centralization was reversed by the decision to reorganize the CPS into 42 local areas, each coterminous with a local police force; second, an inquiry into the operation of the CPS was set up, headed by Sir Iain Glidewell, a retired appeal court judge. The report, published in June 1998, confirmed that the 1993 reorganization of the Service had been a mistake and had resulted in an over-bureaucratized and over-centralized management structure which diverted too many resources from the core activity of conducting prosecutions. The authors of the report estimated that the top 400 CPS lawyers spent less than a third of their time on casework and advocacy. They also expressed their concern that the highest discontinuance rates were for charges of violence against the person and criminal damage and the lowest for motoring offences.

The Glidewell team recommended that cases of downgrading should be examined by the CPS Inspectorate during visits to CPS units and that a single integrated unit to assemble and manage case files should be created, bringing together the present police administration support units and those parts of the CPS dealing with file preparation and review. They emphasized the importance of devolving power and responsibility to the local areas and the need for a rigorous and effective system of accountability. The government welcomed the report, announced that Barbara Mills would be standing down before her contract expires in 1999 and that a new chief executive is to start work

on shifting power from the London headquarters to the local prosecutors (*Guardian*, 2 June 1998). It is to be hoped that as a consequence of
these changes, the CPS will become more open to scrutiny and more
responsive to criticisms of its performance than has been the case in
the past. (See Review of the Crown Prosecution Service (The Glidewell
Report) 1998.)

## Conclusion

In this chapter we have identified two major forces at work within the
criminal justice system, contributing to the extremely high attrition
rate in cases of rape and sexual assault. The first is the police practice
of 'no criming' a high proportion of cases and the second is the
decison-making processes within the Crown Prosecution Service,
involving high levels of 'discontinuance' and 'downgrading'. This is
not, of course, the whole picture, as the fate of those cases that do go
to trial has a decisive impact on the rest of the criminal justice system.
When the police weed out the 'hopeless' cases, they are second-
guessing how the CPS would react to those cases. When the CPS
lawyers discontinue a number of cases that the police would have liked
to see pursued, they are anticipating what would happen if those cases
went to court.

Despite the falling away of so many cases, by no means all those
that do reach court result in a conviction. In our study, 43 of the 71
cases that were heard at court resulted in a conviction, but the majority
of these were cases of indecent assault disposed of in the magistrates'
court. Twelve defendants (involving eleven cases, as in one case there
were two defendants) were given non-custodial sentences. In two cases
suspended sentences were given, one of three months and the other of
twelve months and there were two conditional discharges. Two
community service orders were given, one of 100 hours and the other
of 200 hours, leaving one offender who was bound over for six months
and five offenders for whom financial penalties alone were used,
composed of fines, costs and compensation, involving sums of
between £100 and £330 in each case.

Leaving aside the three defendants who were detained under the
Mental Health Act, in 29 cases custodial sentences were given, ranging
from one month to life imprisonment. In seven of these cases, the
offenders received seven years or more, indicating that if all the hurdles
to a conviction can be overcome, the courts are prepared to recognize
the seriousness of sexual crimes. All seven cases involved rape or

attempted rape and in one case buggery; one involved two suspects, who each received seven year sentences.

At the outset of their account of police and prosecution decision-making, McConville *et al.* (1991) explain how, as a result of undertaking their research, they have come to understand the criminal justice system as a process, rather than a system, in which the apparently discrete stages overlap in important ways, 'so that the overall effect is larger than the sum of the parts' (ibid. 1). Despite this insight, they see the police as largely retaining the upper hand in relation to the prosecution process, so that the exercise of police discretion in the early stages of a reported crime is crucial in shaping the suspect population. It is the police who make the key decisions in relation to 'No Further Action', informal warnings and cautions and it is the police who decide whether or not to consult the CPS before taking these decisions. According to McConville *et al.*, the CPS makes no attempt to get behind police accounts or provide alternatives to them, so that the CPS 'success rate' is very much a product of the police arrest and charge process.

This analysis stands in sharp contrast to the vitriolic attack on the CPS by David Rose (1996a and b). He seems to suggest that the CPS has plenty of room to manoeuvre but that it fails to use its power effectively in the interests of justice. Could it be that there is a coincidence of interests here, whereby both the police and the CPS are preoccupied with success rates rather than with due process considerations? As Sanders (1994) argues, adversarial demands on the police are stronger than justicial demands; once the police have decided that a suspect is guilty, the priority becomes the construction of a watertight case. Similarly, the pressures on the CPS to use 'winnability' as a criterion when screening cases, rather than the 'truth', is overwhelming; so that for the CPS also, the adversarial imperative is stronger than the investigative imperative.

Some 100,000 cases are prosecuted in Crown Courts every year. In more than three-quarters of these, the defendants plead guilty and of the remainder more than half are convicted, with only 10 per cent resulting in acquittals (*The Times*, 15 September 1995). As we shall see in Chapter 4, the pattern of convictions in cases of rape is very different from this and can only partially be explained by focusing on the work of the police and the CPS. The decisions made by judges and juries are a crucial part of the equation. The criminal justice system is indeed a process, so that decisions made at each stage have a profound impact on decisions made at earlier points in the process. For so long as the difficulties of securing a conviction in rape trials persist, the high attrition rate will also persist. Given that it is well nigh impossible to construct a 'watertight' case as far as rape is concerned, the police will continue to reject a high proportion of cases involving interpersonal violence, particularly 'domestic' cases which have no immediate public order implications and in which the victim is 'non-influential' (McConville *et al.* 1991: 34). Nor does the CPS have any reason to challenge such decisions as it too will regard these as the 'weak' and difficult cases. This means that the majority of cases selected for further action will be those that conform most closely to the stereotypical view of the 'classic' rape, a view shared by all the major players in the criminal justice system, including the police, the CPS and the courts.

Behind all the mutual recriminations about the handling of rape and sexual assault cases, the dominant discourse on male and female sexuality, shared by most police officers, lawyers, magistrates, judges and juries, gives rise to the myth of false allegations and to misunderstandings around the notion of consent. Despite demands from women's groups for a radical reform of the way in which sexual assault trials are conducted, supported from time to time by the media in the wake of a case in which the complainant has faced a particularly gruelling ordeal, very little changes. There is a serious mismatch between the conception of crime as an offence against the state, in which the victim is merely a witness in the service of the state, and the reality of the key role that the witness in a sexual assault case plays at every stage of the proceedings. Until this is successfully challenged and the need for a fundamental reshaping of the trial process acknowledged, minor procedural changes are unlikely to have much of an impact on attrition rates. In Chapter 4, we will take a closer look at the cases most likely to fall away, in order to throw more light on the myths prevalent in the dominant discourse on rape and sexual assault.

# 4   The decriminalization of rape?

According to statistics produced by the Home Office, in 1985 24 per cent of the cases recorded by the police in England and Wales as rape resulted in a conviction. In numerical terms, 1,842 crimes of rape were recorded but only 450 of these resulted in a guilty verdict. We know from information provided by rape crisis centres and academic researchers that the vast majority of women who have been raped do not report to the police (see Chapter 1) and we also know from Chapter 3 that a high proportion of rapes that are reported are not recorded as crimes. Already then, the figure of 1,842 rapes occurring in 1985 seems likely to be a gross underestimation of the true incidence of this crime and yet a further 1,392 of these cases fell away, giving an attrition rate of 76 per cent.

Since 1985, there has been a steady increase in the number of cases recorded as rape, so that by 1994 the number had increased almost threefold and 5,039 cases of rape were recorded. The number of convictions, however, was almost identical to that in 1985 (460 as compared to 450); in other words, the conviction rate had dropped dramatically to nine per cent, i.e. an attrition rate of 91 per cent. By 1996 the number of recorded rapes had risen to 5,930 and 576 defendants were found guilty, giving an attrition rate of 90 per cent.[1]

These figures highlight the paradox that more women are coming forward to report rape, encouraged to do so by the more sympathetic treatment they expect to receive from the police and yet the number of men convicted annually of this crime has changed very little. In percentage terms, the proportion of cases resulting in a conviction has shrunk almost to vanishing point. The explanation for this seems to lie in the fact that a steadily increasing proportion of reported rapes do not conform to the stereotypical rape scenario. More of the women reporting nowadays are raped by men they know, often in their own homes, and these are precisely the cases where it is most difficult to secure a conviction.

Despite the lifting of the marital rape exemption, convictions for this particular form of rape are relatively rare, unless the rape is accompanied by extreme levels of violence (Lees 1997b: chapter 6). Marital rape represents one end of a continuum of rape. At the opposite end there is stranger rape, an unexpected attack in an isolated public place by one or more men not previously known to the victim. It is this scenario which resonates with the dominant discourse on rape; the police, the CPS and the courts all feel more comfortable when dealing with stranger rape as the issues seem clear cut. The more contentious issues, regarding such considerations as whether or not the woman consented to intercourse but then changed her mind, or the relevance of previous sexual encounters between her and the rapist, can be avoided.

The trend towards an increasing proportion of reported rapes falling into the 'non-stranger' category was already in evidence during the first half of the 1980s. Lloyd and Walmsley's Home Office study (1989), which was restricted to convicted rapists, and related to a time period prior to the creation of the CPS, seemed to indicate an increased willingness on the part of the courts to convict in cases of non-stranger rape. Lloyd and Walmsley compared the figures on rape convictions in 1985 with the figures for 1973, which had already been analysed in an earlier Home Office study, published by Walmsley and White in 1979. They found a substantial increase in the number of recorded rapes between these two dates. Although there was a fall in the proportion of rapes that resulted in a conviction, there was also a clear shift in the profile of convicted offenders. Whereas in 1973, 47 per cent of convicted rapists were strangers to their victims, by 1985 this had fallen to 39 per cent. The percentage of convicted rapists who were casual acquaintances of the women they attacked had also fallen, although less dramatically, from 39 per cent to 31 per cent.

It was in the third category of 'intimate', where women were raped by relatives, friends or ex-partners, that the biggest change had occurred, so that by 1985 30 per cent of convicted rapists fell into this category, accounting for 67 per cent of the rise in rape convictions between the two dates. Lloyd and Walmsley comment that the most striking finding is the increase in intimates convicted of raping their victim indoors. They suggest that the changes may reflect 'a different attitude on the part of victims (a greater willingness to go to the police), the police (a greater willingness to investigate and prosecute) or the courts (a greater willingness to convict) in respect of offences committed by intimates' (Lloyd and Walmsley 1989: 45).

Does this mean that the profile of convicted rapists is beginning to resemble more closely the profile of rapists in general; that the shape of the part of the iceberg that we see most clearly (convicted rapists) is the same as the part that we see less clearly or not all (unconvicted and unreported rapists)? If there was a tentative move in this direction in the early 1980s, our evidence suggests that the increasingly timid prosecution policies of the police and the Crown Prosecution Service since 1986, in reaction to the high acquittal rate in cases of non-stranger rape, have effectively brought this development to a halt.

Lloyd and Walmsley refer to a second, complementary study undertaken at the same time as theirs and based on a sample of recorded cases of rape, again focusing on the year 1985 but this time including cases that did not lead to a conviction. This study, published in 1992 (Grace *et al.*), makes it possible to assess more carefully the similarities and differences between cases in which a conviction was secured and cases in which it was not. It also provides a useful point of comparison with our own research, relating as it does to a time period immediately prior to the setting up of the CPS. It is important to bear in mind that the Home Office research was based on a national study of England and Wales, excluding the Metropolitan Police District, whereas our research involved an in-depth study of one London Borough.

For ease of comparison with Grace *et al.* (1992) and other studies, we will be concerned in this chapter solely with the 109 cases reported as rape and attempted rape in our study, excluding the 192 cases reported as indecent assault. In terms of the overall attrition process, the 1992 Home Office study provides a useful summary of the various stages at which cases fall away. Table 4.1 reproduces this information and compares it with the attrition rate for the 109 cases included in our research. The first major difference is the much higher 'no criming' rate evident in our study. As we explained in Chapter 1, this is due to the inclusion of cases 'no crimed' during the first month after the crime report was received, excluded from the research by Grace *et al.* (1992) because it was based on the monthly statistical returns to the Home Office. The rates of detection were higher in the Home Office study but so were the rates of cautioning. We found no cases of rape or attempted rape in which the suspect was let off with a caution.

Although the percentage of cases in which the police took no further action (NFA) is higher than in the Home Office study (20 per cent as compared with 16 per cent in our research), there is an additional layer of decision-making in the present study, in the shape of

*Table 4.1* Overall attrition rate: the Home Office study and the present study compared

| | No. | Attrition | No. | %* |
|---|---|---|---|---|
| *The Home Office study, Grace et al. (1992)* | | | | |
| Initially recorded as an offence | 335 | | | |
| Finally recorded as an offence | 255 | 'No crimed' | 80 | 24 |
| Detected | 223 | Undetected | 32 | 33 |
| Proceeded with by police | 178 | No further action | 45 | 47 |
| Prosecuted | 170 | Cautioned | 8 | 49 |
| Convicted for an offence | 136 | Not guilty/discharged | 34 | 59 |
| Convicted for rape/attempted rape | 89 | Convicted for a lesser offence | 47 | 73 |
| | | | | |
| *Our study, rape/attempted rape only* | | | | |
| Total rapes reported | 109 | | | |
| Recorded as an offence | 60 | 'No crimed' | 49 | 45 |
| Detected | 44 | Undetected | 16 | 60 |
| To CPS | 37 | NFA by police | 7 | 66 |
| To court | 30 | NFA by CPS | 7 | 72 |
| Convicted for an offence | 12 | Not guilty/discharged | 18 | 89 |
| Convicted for rape/attempted rape | 9 | Convicted for a lesser offence | 3 | 92 |

*Note*: * cumulative

the Crown Prosecution Service, which added a further 16 per cent to the NFA category, so that 32 per cent (14 out of 44) of the detected cases did not proceed to court. Despite this higher rate of attrition in the earlier stages, a smaller proportion of cases going to court resulted in a conviction, 40 per cent as compared with 80 per cent of cases. Putting aside the 'no criming' figures, which are not comparable, and expressing these findings as an overall attrition rate, we find that in the Grace study 53 per cent of the 'crimed' cases resulted in a conviction for rape or a lesser offence, whereas in our study only 20 per cent of the 'crimed' cases had this outcome. If the 'no crimed' cases are included in our study, the overall conviction rate falls to 11 per cent.

These findings are in line with the Home Office statistics presented at the beginning of this chapter, indicating a substantial rise in attrition rates between 1985 and the mid-1990s. What the statistics do not reveal is the factors associated with attrition; what it is that determines whether or not a case proceeds through all stages of the criminal justice process, culminating in a conviction. The study by Grace *et al.* (1992) attempted to answer this question by identifying some of the factors associated with attrition. Referring to a study by

Williams (1984) which lists the factors that most researchers have identified as strongly associated with an individual's decision to report a rape as race, age, marital status and relationship to the rapist, they claim that these same factors are also correlated with attrition once a rape has been reported. In fact, the list of variables explored in their report does not coincide precisely with the factors mentioned by Williams. Grace *et al.* introduce additional factors such as the location of the attack and the degree of violence involved. They are silent on the question of race, except for a table in an appendix showing that 75 per cent of the suspects were white and 15 per cent were Afro-Caribbean.

They find that cases involving younger (under 16) and older (over 50) women were more likely to result in a conviction than those involving women from other age groups; cases involving single women were more likely to be 'crimed' and to result in a conviction; cases in which there was evidence of violence and injury were also more likely to lead to a conviction. In our study we had no information on marital status and the information on the ages of victims was incomplete, but we can confirm that force was used in eight of the nine cases in our study which resulted in a conviction for rape. The most interesting findings in the Home Office study from the point of view of our research are those relating to the relationship between complainant and suspect, although direct comparisons are difficult, because of the different definitions used in the two studies to identify this relationship.

## The relationship between complainant and suspect

Both studies use the three categories 'stranger', 'acquaintance' and 'intimate', but the Home Office study uses a broader definition of an intimate relationship, including relatives, friends and work colleagues, whereas we have restricted this category to relationships that have a sexual dimension, such as ex-husband, ex-boyfriend and ex-cohabitee.[2] The definition of 'acquaintance' used by Grace *et al.* also differs from ours in that it includes a category 'acquaintance within 24 hours' (and one case of hitchhiking), which in our study has been subsumed within the 'stranger' category. In both studies, the 'acquaintance' group embraces a wide range of relationships; in our study, it ranges from 'knew by sight' to 'family friend' and in the Home Office study from 'known vaguely' to 'acquainted prior to 24 hours'. The decision as to which definitions are more appropriate will depend on the kind of analysis that is required.

Grace *et al.* report that 30 per cent of the cases included in their study fell into the category of stranger rapes, 35 per cent involved acquaintances and 35 per cent intimates. Our narrower definition of 'intimate' and broader definition of 'stranger' gave us a breakdown of 51 per cent stranger rapes, 32 per cent acquaintance rapes and 17 per cent intimate rapes.

### The pattern of 'no criming'

The Home Office study reported similar 'no criming' rates for all three groups, with a very slightly higher rate for the 'intimate' category. In our study, which included reported rapes 'no crimed' in the first month, clear differences were apparent between the three groups, so that 35 per cent of stranger rapes were 'no crimed', whereas this was the case for 51 per cent of acquaintance rapes and 61 per cent of rapes involving intimates. In other words, when all the 'no crimed' cases are included, from the moment of reporting onwards, it becomes clear that the attrition rate is already impacting more severely on cases where some form of relationship between the complainant and the suspect existed prior to the alleged attack. The police are both anticipating what will happen at later stages in the process and giving expression to their own stereotypical views on what constitutes rape, views which reflect those prevalent in the wider society.

Although the Grace *et al.* study found no significant differences in the 'no criming' rates for each of the three categories, they did find that the reasons for 'no criming' showed a distinctive pattern. Reports of rapes by strangers were most likely to be 'no crimed' because the allegation was considered false or malicious, whereas acquaintance rapes were most often 'no crimed' because the woman withdrew her complaint. This confirms our finding, that complaint-initiated withdrawals were much more common in cases of non-stranger rape (see Chapter 3).

Grace *et al.* find that the intimate category was much more evenly spread, with 39 per cent of women withdrawing their complaint, 27 per cent categorized as false allegations, 15 per cent of cases in which the women were unwilling to testify and 15 per cent marked as 'insufficient evidence'. This contrasts with our findings, which show that all the 'no crimed' cases in the intimate category were complainant-initiated withdrawals, in which the complainant withdrew or refused to substantiate the allegation, leading us to conclude that the greater the degree of intimacy, the more likely it is that the suspect may exert pressure to ensure that the case is dropped. The less clear-cut findings in the Home Office study may be due to the rather 'mixed bag' of relationships included in their 'intimate' category.

### The pattern of convictions

Not surprisingly, in both studies attacks by strangers had the lowest detection rate of the three groups. Leaving aside those cases in which the suspect was not identified, Grace *et al.* find that cases involving strangers were more likely to go to court and to result in a conviction for rape; that cases involving intimates were the least likely to proceed to a prosecution and that cases involving acquaintances were the most likely to result in an acquittal. This gives them a conviction rate of 58 per cent for detected stranger rapes, 41 per cent for rapes involving acquaintances and 43 per cent for the intimate category.

The equivalent percentages in our research were 45 per cent for stranger rape, falling to 30 per cent if we exclude cases where the conviction was for a lesser offence; 24 per cent for acquaintance rape, falling to 18 per cent when one case was reversed on appeal; and 0 per cent in the case of rapes involving intimates. However, as the total number of convictions for rape and attempted rape resulting from the 109 cases did not even run into double figures (see Table 4.1), it is more meaningful to express these findings numerically. Of the 12 cases of stranger rape that reached court, 9 resulted in a conviction, 6 of these for rape and 3 for a lesser offence. Of the 14 cases of acquaintance rape that reached court, only 4 resulted in a conviction and one of these was reversed on appeal. Of the 5 cases of rape by intimates that reached court, not one secured a conviction. These figures show conclusively that the closer the relationship between the complainant and the defendant, the greater the difficulty in securing a conviction. They also provide a vivid illustration of the 'knock-back' effect, so that decisions made in court have a powerful influence on decision-making at earlier stages in the criminal justice process.

We have already commented on the lower overall success rate in our research compared with that found in the earlier study, but it is also interesting to note the different pattern of acquittals in the two studies. In the Home Office research it was the acquaintance category that exhibited the highest acquittal rate, whereas in our study, although the acquittal rate in cases of acquaintance rape was high (10 of the 14 cases reaching court), the intimate category achieved a 100 per cent acquittal rate, with none of the five cases reaching court securing a conviction. Grace *et al.* comment in relation to their findings that a defence of consent seems more likely to succeed in the acquaintance category due to the circumstances surrounding the attack.

Corroboration is very often difficult in rape cases and if incidents are open to interpretation as consensual, the likelihood of conviction falls. The case for the defence will almost always hinge on whether or not the defendant consented to intercourse. It is easy to infer that this is the case if there is a lack of physical evidence and if the woman's behaviour can be presented as blameworthy in some respect. In such cases, it appears that the odds are continually against the case being detected, proceeded with and resulting in a conviction for rape. It is far more likely that the case will be subject to the process of attrition.

(Grace *et al.* 1992)

This issue is vividly illustrated by the case in our research in which a conviction for rape was quashed on appeal. A police officer gave us the following details. A young woman had locked herself out of her flat on a hot summer's day and went to a friend's house in order to telephone her boyfriend. She failed to make contact, but a young male acquaintance offered her a bed for the night. According to her account, she awoke to find him on top of her and she was then raped. She ran from the flat in a distressed state and immediately reported the rape to the police.

At the trial, the judge allowed character witnesses to be called on behalf of the defendant and also permitted the complainant to be cross-examined about three sexual incidents in her past, involving men other than the accused. Section 2 of the Sexual Offences (Amendment) Act 1976 was intended to control the use of sexual history evidence, but the decision in each case is left to the discretion of the judge (see Chapter 1). In this case, the jury was unable to reach a verdict and a retrial was ordered, so that the complainant had to endure the trauma of the trial a second time. On this occasion, a woman judge allowed the character evidence and one of the sexual incidents to be heard, but disallowed the other two as irrelevant. During the hearing, friends of the defendant referred to the complainant as 'a tart and an easy lay' and as 'behaving like a frustrated actress'. Despite this sustained attack on the complainant's moral character, the jury found the defendant, a Mr Bogie, guilty.

Mr Bogie appealed, claiming that the trial was unfair because of the judge's refusal to allow the full sexual history evidence to be heard. The Court of Appeal agreed and quashed the conviction, referring to the complainant as 'an unusually neurotic and unbalanced girl who was capable of making up allegations of sexual misconduct for no good reason' (quoted in Temkin 1993). Unlike the defendant, there is no-one to speak on behalf of the complainant; she is merely there as witness for the state and because the state has no need of protection, she is left exposed. When a judge attempts to provide some protection by controlling the introduction of irrelevant sexual history evidence as the law intended, the conviction is quashed.[3]

### Further Home Office research

Yet another Home Office research project on the processing of rape cases was started during 1997, reflecting official concern with the falling conviction rate in such cases. At the time of writing, only the interim report from this research was available (Harris 1997) and it largely confirms the trends in attrition rates that we have identified in earlier research. Based on 309 cases of rape reported to three police forces since February 1996, it reveals that the tendency for women to report attacks by men they know has continued. Only 8 per cent of the rapes analysed in the Harris study so far were stranger rapes (compared with 30 per cent in the Grace *et al.* (1992) study), whereas 50 per cent were rapes by intimates (compared with 35 per cent). The 'no criming' rate is comparable at 23 per cent, but the percentage of cases in which the police decide to take no further action has risen substantially, constituting 37 per cent of the total (113 of the 309 reported cases) and demonstrating the influence of the CPS role on police practice in forwarding cases for prosecution (Harris 1997). As a result of this dramatic rise in the proportion of cases indicated as NFA by the police, a mere 24 per cent of cases reached court in the later study, compared to the 50 per cent reported by Grace *et al.* (1992).

On the basis of these interim findings, Harris concludes that the cases most likely to drop out of the process are those involving adult women over 35 years old, those where there is no evidence of violence or injury and those where there were greater degrees of consensual contact between the complainant and the suspect prior to the rape.

### Consenting to rape

Almost half the cases categorized in the Home Office study as 'acquaintance' rape were where the complainant 'vaguely' knew her attacker or had met him within 24 hours. Yet if such cases are catego- rized as 'stranger' rather than 'acquaintance' rapes, which we would argue is more logical, the balance between the two categories would not have changed since 1985. In our research 51 per cent fell into the category we designated as 'stranger' compared to a mere 8 per cent in the Harris study.

There is a further reason why including 'met within 24 hours' as a 'stranger' relationship seems a more accurate form of categorization. It throws some light on the paradox of why advances in DNA technology should have coincided with a sharp decline rather than an increase in the conviction rate. In the 1990s a National Home Office Major Enquiry System (HOMES) was set up whereby DNA information can be downloaded so that offences such as rapes, murders or other crimes can be linked up. These advances have had two effects. Firstly, it is now far more possible to identify rapes which occur in different police authorities. Secondly, it undermines the defence of 'identification' where the defendant argues that he was not the assailant. This means that the classic defence of the 'stranger' rapist – that it was not he who committed the offence – is disproved by forensic evidence.

The decline rather than the increase in the conviction rate which one might expect may be due to serial rapists adapting their tactics in the face of DNA advances. They may well have realized that a defence of 'consent' where they mimic the stereotypical 'date rape' scenario is far more likely to lead to successful acquittals. Indeed in the *Dispatches* (1994) research undertaken by Lees (1997a), three serial rapists were identified who used exactly such tactics and had been acquitted again and again. One man, convicted as a stereotypical 'stranger' rapist who had attacked a woman with a knife, progressed to adopting the more subtle 'chatting up' tactic before isolating his victim and raping her. Since adopting these tactics, he had stood trial and been acquitted four times. Another defendant had stood trial four times before absconding without trace before a fifth trial. The third defendant was reported for rape by eight different young women totally unconnected with one another. The tactics he used were similar in all cases. He went to night clubs and persuaded young women to get into his car on some pretext, and would then hold them captive driving them at speed into the country in order to rape them. Yet in only one of these cases was he convicted when his barrister made the mistake of putting him in the witness box. The *Dispatches* research demonstrated why such rapists had a very high chance of acquittal.

The extreme difficulty of securing a conviction in such cases is due to seeing the victim as contributing to her own downfall by behaving inappropriately, by being in a nightclub at all or by wearing what is described as 'provocative clothing'. The idea that perfectly normal behaviour can be seen as provocation to assault, encourages serial rape, with the rapists deliberately adopting a *modus operandi*, such as targeting young women in night clubs, confident that they will go unpunished time and time again (*Dispatches* 1994, Lees 1997b: chapter 6). An added problem is that a drug known as Rohypnol, available on the black market, is being acquired by men for the purpose of spiking young women's drinks in clubs before assaulting them. It causes temporary memory loss while supposedly heightening sexual desire and has the added advantage that it leaves no traces in the body only a relatively short time after it has been consumed. This development could increase the attractiveness of this form of criminal activity without in any way increasing the conviction rate. In the United States it has been implicated in more than 500 assaults (see Brooks 1998).

It seems likely therefore that a significant proportion of men who are being categorized as having committed 'date rape', where they have met their victim within 24 hours of the assault, are actually serial rapists who know how to play the system and go out of their way to establish a brief acquaintance with the victim – acutely aware of how much it will help the defence (see *Guardian*, Analysis supplement, 17 June 1998). The implication here is clearly that this type of rape is of a totally different order from 'real' rape and is due to men misreading signals and being confused. In an article by Alan Travis entitled 'Alarm over "Date Rapes" (*Guardian* 16th June 1998) the Home Office was reported to have suggested that the decline in the conviction rate could be due to the fact that 'half of all rapes are being reported as "date rapes" – committed by boyfriends, former partners or close friends – compared to 35 per cent a decade ago'. It would be far more accurate to categorize attackers who have met their victims on the same day as strangers. Examining the figures with that in mind, there has not been a change in the proportion of stranger rapes between 1985 and 1996.

Another type of rape characterized as 'date rape', as in the *Guardian* article of 18th June, is by an ex-boyfriend. Such attacks occur when the relationship has ended and often involve serious injuries. 'Date rape' where the couple make a pre-arrangement to go out and where the woman is raped occurs far less frequently but these are often the cases which attract a great deal of press publicity.

As Lees (1997a) shows in her monitoring of cases that appeared at the Old Bailey in 1994, acquaintance rapists are often serial rapists who plan their assaults carefully. Their tactics include picking up young women and discovering as much as they can about them before raping them, with a view to using this information in court as evidence of a strong relationship. Such men know how to use the judicial system to their own advantage and are acquitted again and again.

Attrition rates of some 90 per cent, rising to almost 100 per cent in cases of non-stranger rape, would seem to justify the deliberately provocative title of this chapter, suggesting that we are indeed witnessing the decriminalization of rape. By 'losing' almost all of those cases of reported rape in which there was some prior acquaintance between the suspect and the complainant, the criminal justice system is in effect condoning such crimes. However, only if the conviction rate for rape were to slump to zero would the claim of total decriminalization stand up. In the meantime, it is worth turning the question around in order to examine more closely the tiny handful of cases that survive the criminal justice obstacle course in order to secure a conviction for rape at the end of the process.

## Race and sexual and domestic assault

We know that criminalization is most likely to occur in cases of stranger rape, particularly where there is evidence of violence and injury, but there may be other ways in which these cases are untypical. Specifically, there is a growing body of research evidence pointing to the existence of discriminatory practices within the criminal justice system, resulting in higher conviction rates and harsher penalties for offences involving suspects from minority racial and ethnic groups. This is a highly sensitive issue which many researchers are reluctant to comment on. As we saw earlier, Grace *et al.* (1992) collected data on ethnicity but presented no detailed analysis, mainly because the records on ethnicity were incomplete. Similarly, Lorna Smith (1989) found that the ethnicity of suspects was recorded in only 365 of the 507 cases in her sample, but she concluded that even if it is assumed that all the offenders for whom racial origins were not recorded were white, African Caribbean offenders were over-represented in the figures of recorded rapes in both Islington and Lambeth. As one possible explanation for this over-representation, she suggests that black women may be more likely to report rape than white women and quotes some figures from the National Crime Survey in the United States which support this assertion, particularly in relation to the reporting of non-stranger rape.

As Daly and Stephens (1995) point out, very little is known about black women's experiences of victimization. The most thorough study of black women and domestic violence, *The Hidden Struggle*, was carried out by Amina Mama (1989) in London. She conducted interviews with 100 black women between November 1987 and October 1988 and found that 53 per cent of the women interviewed had had contact with the police. This is considerably higher than that found in other studies concerned with the incidence of male violence. It would seem to confirm the findings of a study by Jayne Mooney (1993) that African Caribbean women have lower tolerance levels to domestic violence and are also more likely to report domestic violence to the police than white women. However, it is important to note that other minority racial and ethnic groups, including Asian and African women who might be particularly vulnerable to persecution under immigration laws, had extremely low reporting rates (Mooney 1993). Also, in many of the cases documented in the Amina Mama study, neighbours or friends had made the call.

In comparing the findings, it is important to take into account the different methodologies employed. Mama (1989) obtained her sample through the Women's Aid network and all the women interviewed had been subjected to severe degrees of cruelty which 'rendered the definitional problems around more borderline cases irrelevant' (Mama 1989: 40). Mooney's sample, on the other hand, was based on a randomized community study and takes as its starting point a very wide definition of domestic violence to include 'mental cruelty, threats, sexual abuse, physical violence and any form of controlling behaviour' (1993: 8). Similarly, a study of sexual violence by Kelly (1988) specifically sets out to explore violence as a continuum, not in order to create a hierarchy of abuse, but in order to demonstrate how women can make sense of their own experiences by showing how 'typical' and 'aberrant' male behaviour shade one into the other (1988: 75).

A more recent study by Kelly *et al.* (1998), based on the Duluth crisis intervention project in the United States, is an evaluation of a pilot project based in Islington known as Domestic Violence Matters. It involved civilians working alongside the police in police stations. Kelly found that 21 per cent of the women worked with were black and a further ten per cent were from ethnic minorities, particularly Turkish and Irish; these percentages are considerably higher than the black and ethnic minority populations of the borough. Referring to other studies documenting the deep distrust of the police on the part of certain sections of ethnic minority communities, Kelly *et al.* comment that this distrust appears to coexist with a frequent resort to the police by some members of those communities. They surmise that these women may be particularly isolated from other sources of help such as kin and community (Kelly *et al.* 1998). In contrast to this suggestion, black students in Sue Lees' seminar at the University of North London described black women as having very good networks to support each other in calling the police when subjected to violence. They also believed that the predominantly white police force was more prepared to take action against black men than against white men.

The relationship between race and rape is a particularly sensitive issue in the United States because of the history of lynching. During the slavery period, rape involving a black offender and a white victim was treated extremely harshly, involving the death penalty or castration. Although most lynchings did not involve the accusation of sexual assault, the cry of rape became a populist justification for mob attacks on black men. In those states where it was illegal for white men to rape white women, the penalties were less severe and the rape of black women by white or black men was legal (Wriggins 1983). After the Civil War, rape statutes were made race-neutral, but in practice the myth of the 'black rapist' was still prevalent, feeding off racist ideology (Davis 1981).

In the post-Civil War period, the very threat of lynch mobs would be enough to ensure a conviction in the courts, particularly as the jury were permitted to consider 'social conditions and customs founded upon racial differences'; in other words, to assume that black men wanted to rape white women but that a white woman would never consent to sex with a black man (Wriggins 1983: 111). Between 1930 and 1967, 36 per cent of the black men who were convicted of raping white women were executed, so that 89 per cent of the men executed for rape were black (Wriggins 1983). It is still the case in the US that black men convicted of raping white women receive longer prison sentences than other rape defendants, thus contributing to the false notion of rape as a violent crime between strangers where the perpetrator is black and the victim white.

Research evidence from the United States and Britain indicates that most sexual crimes are intra-racial, i.e. the victims and suspects are members of the same racial or ethnic group (LaFree 1980, 1989). However, as one moves further away from the commission of the crime towards the point at which a conviction is secured, inter-racial sexual crimes, particularly those involving black male suspects and white female complainants, appear to be more common, as other cases fall away. LaFree found that inter-racial crimes where the victim is white and the assailant black are more likely to reach court and secure a conviction. Similarly, the American National Crime Survey 1984 found that reporting was race-related with more white women reporting rapes by black males (23 per cent of the total) than black women reporting rapes by white males (8 per cent) (see also Bourque 1989). The preponderance of studies of black ghettoes may be one reason for this finding; see for example Amir's study (1971) where 80 per cent of assailants and victims were black but the study was conducted in a predominantly black neighbourhood.

In Britain there has been little research into the connections between race and sexual crimes. Smith's Home Office study (1989a) was the first designed with a view to developing a profile of rape. The cases were drawn from two London Boroughs selected because of their high levels of recorded rape but also containing large ethnic minority populations. Her findings confirm those from American research, indicating that most sexual attacks are intra-racial. She found that 96 per cent of African Caribbean victims were raped by African Caribbean men and that four-fifths of them were raped by men they knew. She also found that 'the ethnicity of the offender was not a factor which influenced the decision to record a reported offence as a crime' (Smith 1989a: 20) but, as we have seen, many of the records did not specify the race of the offender or victim.

Against this background, we turn to the findings of our own research. Information on the racial origins of both suspects and complainants was available in only 86 of the 109 reported cases of rape and attempted rape. Among the cases in which the information was missing, either for the suspect, the complainant or both, were some which did make progress through the criminal justice system and some where the complainant and suspect were known to each other. This means that the absence of information is due to sloppy recording practices and could also mean that the information we do have is inaccurate, a suspicion confirmed by the experience of Paul Myers, an Afro-Caribbean press officer with the Metropolitan Police. He describes how, after being stopped and searched for no reason, he obtained a copy of his search record. His ethnic group had been entered as 'Asian' and his close-cropped curly hair described as 'flicked back' (Myers 1997; see also the confusion over racial characteristics in the case discussed above, in Chapter 3).

Seventy-three (85 per cent) of the women reporting rape or attempted rape in our study were recorded as white and only thirteen (15 per cent) as non-white: nine were classified as black, three as Asian and one as Chinese.[4] Six of the cases involving ethnic minority women were stranger rapes, five were acquaintance rapes and only two involved intimates. These findings do not support the view that Afro-Caribbean women are more likely to report violence to the police, particularly by men known to them; five of the nine complainants classified as black were reporting stranger-rapes.

Turning to the ethnicity of suspects, like Lorna Smith, we found a higher percentage of non-white suspects than would be expected from the ethnic composition of the area: 48 (56 per cent) of the suspects were white and 38 (44 per cent) were non-white. Twenty-nine of the non-white suspects were classified as black, eight as Asian and one as Chinese. In contrast to Lorna Smith's findings however, our figures do show a relationship between ethnicity and the practice of 'no criming', so that whereas 37 per cent (14) of the reported crimes involving non-white suspects were 'no crimed', 48 per cent (23) of those involving white suspects were 'no crimed'. In other words, white defendants were more likely to drop out of the system at the recording stage.

Clearly, it would be unwise to jump to conclusions merely on the basis of these figures, but on further analysis, it becomes clear that non-white defendants are more often facing accusations of inter-racial rape and these are the cases that are more likely to be reported and to be 'crimed' by the police, particularly when they involve white complainants and non-white defendants. Whereas 44 white suspects were accused of intra-racial rape, this was true of only seven non-white suspects and the 'no criming' rate for both these groups was roughly 50 per cent. Turning to accusations of inter-racial rape, the tables are reversed, with 11 white suspects falling into this category and experiencing a 'no criming' rate of 73 per cent and 31 non-white suspects facing the same accusation, but experiencing a much lower 'no criming' rate of 32 per cent. In other words, according to our findings, white women are more likely to report serious sexual assaults by non-white men and these are the cases most likely to be taken forward by the police. As can be seen from Table 4.2, this difference applies both

*Table 4.2* 'Crimed' and 'no crimed' cases of rape and attempted rape by ethnicity and relationship

|  | Stranger | | Acquaintance | | Intimate | | Total | |
|---|---|---|---|---|---|---|---|---|
|  | C | NC | C | NC | C | NC | C | NC |
| Intra-racial (white) | 15 | 7 | 2 | 8 | 5 | 7 | 22 | 22 |
| Intra-racial (non-white) | 1 | 2 | 2 | 1 | 0 | 1 | 3 | 4 |
| Inter-racial involving white suspects | 2 | 1 | 0 | 0 | 1 | 0 | 3 | 1 |
| Inter-racial involving non-white suspects | 13 | 5 | 8 | 4 | 0 | 1 | 21 | 10 |
| Total | 31 | 15 | 12 | 13 | 6 | 9 | 49 | 37 |

*Notes*:
C: crimed
NC: no crimed

to stranger and acquaintance rapes, but not to the intimate category, where almost all the reported cases involved white complainants and white suspects.

From the information available, it would appear that reported cases of rape or attempted rape involving inter-racial attacks are more likely to be 'crimed' than those involving intra-racial attacks and there is no obvious alternative explanation, for example in terms of the different levels of violence reported. However, previous researchers have warned of the dangers of drawing conclusions concerning racial bias on the basis of incomplete evidence; for example, in the absence of information about previous criminal records (see for example Hirsch and Roberts 1997). Any conclusions to be drawn from our findings are therefore necessarily tentative; although we cannot identify other associated variables which would account for the differences, our information is necessarily incomplete.

Turning to the ethnicity of the nine cases in which a conviction was secured, the picture becomes even less clear. Six of the nine were cases of intra-racial rape; in five of these, both the complainant and the defendant were white and in the sixth both were Afro-Caribbean. Of the remaining cases, two involved Afro-Caribbean defendants and white complainants and in the third the defendant was white and the complainant Chinese. With such a high attrition rate, it is difficult to come to any firm conclusion as to what it was that distinguished the nine 'successful' cases from the one hundred that fell away. As we have seen, six of them were stranger rapes, eight involved violence and in three the defendants were black. It is worth noting also that two were 'gang' rapes, each involving two defendants; in one case they were both white and in the other case both of them were black. This information gives us the factors associated with cases that result in a conviction. What it does not explain, however, is why so many other cases sharing these characteristics failed to secure that outcome.

## Gang rape

As we have seen, two of the nine cases in our study which resulted in a conviction were cases of gang rape. In a third case, there was a partial conviction in the sense that one of the defendants was sentenced to six months imprisonment for buggery but was found not guilty of rape; the other defendant was found not guilty on both counts. There is no record of either the age or the ethnicity of the suspects or complainant in this case. The facts recorded in the crime report are as follows:

> Victim answered a knock at the door and found suspects outside (she had known one of them for a couple of weeks). They forced her inside and took it in turns to rape and bugger her. This continued for about one and a half hours before they left.

The suspect, who was not known to the complainant, received the six month sentence. It is not clear why both suspects were acquitted of the rape charge; as the attack occurred in the complainant's home, presumably the defendants claimed that she had invited them in and consented to sex. It would not, of course, be legally possible for her to consent to buggery.

There are two more cases of gang rape among the 109 reported rapes and attempted rapes in our study. Both of them involved black complainants and black suspects. One was discharged at the magistrates' court and the other was 'no crimed' by the police. This second case was a classic 'stranger' rape:

> Victim walked down the road and was grabbed by three suspects who dragged her into a community hallway. Two of them held her down while a third one raped her. Victim reported crime, then has failed to contact or assist police since report.

The records show that she was referred to Victim Support, but there is no indication as to whether or not a meeting with a Victim Support volunteer took place.

The other case was acquaintance rape:

> Victim met suspects in a nightclub and they offered her a lift home. She accepted but was taken to the home of one of the suspects. She was ordered to take her clothes off. When she refused, she was punched in the face. Both men then had full sexual intercourse by force.

This case was discharged when the complainant withdrew her allegation; she was 17.

These two cases raise a number of serious issues that merit further investigation. It would seem that the complainants were unwilling to pursue their cases, either through fear of reprisals or because they could not face the ordeal that lay ahead if the cases went to court. Unfortunately, it is outcomes such as these that in effect convey the message to young men that they can rape with impunity. In two of the nine convictions in our study, other sexual attacks by the defendants were taken into consideration. There is no way of knowing what proportion of the sexual attacks reported to the police are in fact the work of serial rapists.

The study of male rape indicates that here too a significant proportion are by gangs and are even less likely to be reported. Very few cases reach court due to fear of retaliation and the shame and humiliation victims undergo. It is likely that gangs, like individuals, may rape for a variety of reasons. Some may be predominantly homophobic and others may have a racial motive (see Chapter 5).

There is growing evidence of gang rapes involving children, both as victims and perpetrators. In September 1996, eight boys from North London aged 14 to 17 were arrested for the gang rape of a 33-year-old Austrian tourist who had been thrown into a canal. In May 1997 further cases of gang rape involving even younger boys came to light: four 10-year-old boys and a 9 year old were arrested in West London for the alleged rape of a 9-year-old girl in a school toilet during the lunch break. In the same week a boy of 13 appeared before Wolverhampton magistrates charged with raping a 12-year-old girl on a disused railway line and two boys aged 13 and 15 were charged with indecent assault (*Guardian*, 10 May 1997). In January 1998 two 10-year-old boys were charged with rape and two of indecent assault of a classmate in a school toilet (Campbell 1998); all of them were acquitted after the young girl was cross-examined about her past sexual history. Convictions are no easier to achieve in cases involving children under 14 than in other cases (Soothill 1997). It is likely that such cases are the tip of the iceberg and that, possibly due to earlier maturation, sexual violence is becoming a problem in primary schools.

## Conclusion

Table 4.3 provides a summary of the information available from our study on the nine reports of rape or attempted rape that resulted in a conviction. It confirms that a conviction is more likely in cases of stranger rape and in cases where force is used. In two of the convictions involving acquaintances there was a substantial age gap between the complainant and the defendant. In the third case a 13-year-old girl was raped by two teenage boys in a children's home. The one who had held her down was given a conditional discharge while the one who had raped her was given 100 hours community service. This was the only conviction for rape in which the offenders were not sent to prison.

Our findings demonstrate that the most crucial factor determining whether or not a case will result in a conviction is the relationship between the assailant and the complainant. In the case of stranger rape, provided the assailant is identified, and given the availability of DNA evidence, the chances of obtaining a conviction are quite high. However, even in cases possessing all the characteristics of a 'classic' rape, if there has been any kind of verbal communication between the man and the woman prior to the attack, the chances of securing a conviction are considerably reduced. Any previous sexual contact is highly prejudicial; in our study, there was not a single conviction in this category. Lees' (1997b: chapter 6) examination of marital rape appeals indicated that such cases are likely to involve multiple injuries which are suggestive of attempted murder, with the complainant often losing consciousness through strangulation, which is the most common method by which women are murdered. Cases involving marital rape are also likely to receive significantly lower sentences, in breach of the Billam guidelines (see Chapter 1). Rumney (1999), in his analysis of 100 cases of marital rape which were appealed, found that the average sentence for marital rape was less than the average sentence for attempted rape, and that aggravating factors were constantly downplayed.

In this chapter we have criticized the common assumption that the fall in the rate of conviction in rape cases is due to an increase in 'date' or 'acquaintance' rapes. Instead we have argued that as a result of advances in forensic techniques it is no longer worth serial rapists attacking strangers and then pleading not guilty on the grounds that it was not they who committed the offences. Instead they are adapting their tactics to meet this new situation and instead of assaulting their victims anonymously they are entering into communication prior to the assault so that, in the event of being apprehended, they can plead that the victim consented in the knowledge that they will have a good chance of being acquitted. These men are not 'date' rapists who misread signals but plan their rapes carefully and know exactly what they are doing. Therefore we suggest that defendants categorized by the Home Office researchers as 'met within 24 hours' should be more accurately described as stranger rapists rather than acquaintance rapists. This analysis suggests that serial rapists who plan their rapes  carefully are finding it easier than ever to get away with rape in the light of the failure of the Sexual Offences (Amendment) Act 1976 to be implemented.

In Chapter 5, we report on the first study of the ways in which the police deal with reported cases of rape in which the complainants as well as the suspects are men. This will enable us to explore differences and similarities in the police construction of male and female rape and to analyse police recording practices in relation to male rape.

*Table 4.3* Sentences for rape and attempted rape: key characteristics of the nine convictions

| Crime | Sentence | Relationship | Ethnicity C | Ethnicity D | Use or threat of force | Location of crime |
|---|---|---|---|---|---|---|
| Rape | Life +5 years (IA) 3 years (ABH) | stranger | white | white | ABH, buggery | street |
| Rape | 9 years + 6 years (robbery) 2 years (deception) | stranger | white | white | force used | C's home |
| Rape (2 defendants) | 7 years each | strangers (both) | white | white | force used | street |
| Attempted Rape | 8 years | stranger | white | white | knife (scratches) | C's home (break-in) |
| Attempted Rape | 7 years (another rape TIC) | stranger | white | black | cuts + bruises | street |
| Attempted Rape | 3 years youth custody (5 counts of IA TIC) | stranger | white | white | GBH, vaginal bleeding, cuts + bruises | street |
| Rape | 6 years (8 years for buggery) | *acquaintance | oriental | white | ABH, cuts + bruises | C's daughter's home |
| Rape | 6 years | *acquaintance | black | black | no force | party |
| Rape (2 defendants) | (i) conditional discharge (ii) community service order 100 hours | acquaintances | white | black (both) | bruises | C's home (council home) |

*Notes:*
C: complainant
D: defendant
TIC: taken into consideration
* In both these cases, there was a substantial age gap between the complainant and the defendant.

# 5    Male rape: the crime that can now speak its name

In this chapter the police service approach to male sexual assaults on men is explored in relation to consultancy and research undertaken for a Channel 4 *Dispatches* programme, 'Male Rape' (1995). This was commissioned about a year after the success of the 1994 *Dispatches* programme which investigated reasons for the rise in the attrition rate for female rape cases 'Getting Away with Rape'.[1] It also occurred at a time when the law on male attacks was about to change and penetration of the anus was to be classified for the first time as rape. The programme was based on two surveys. The first involved a survey of victims comprising an analysis of 85 questionnaires completed by male victims of rape who contacted researchers by telephone after advertisements were placed in national and local newspapers. For a full report on this research see Lees (1997b). The second survey, based on police records, is reported here. It was one of the first attempts to investigate the police response to reporting of rape of men by men. In the light of the improvement of the treatment of female victims of rape, we were interested in whether the police had adapted similar techniques to deal with male victims of assault

Co-operation was negotiated with the Association of Chief Police Officers and the Police Federation. All 43 police forces in England and Wales were asked if they were willing to complete a fourteen-page questionnaire on all non-consensual buggeries and rape on males, aged 16 and over, reported to them in the previous two years. The questionnaire was designed for the purposes of compiling statistical data only. Most questions involved 'tick boxes'. Questionnaires were completed by the investigating officer in each case, based on crime reports and interviews with victims and suspects. In total 81 questionnaires were received from 15 forces; 60 of these were male rapes including anal penile penetration, as at least one of the indecent acts committed, and 21 related to indecent assaults. The other police forces did not respond so only a minority of police forces took part in the survey. Some were unwilling or unable to co-operate. Others reported that no rapes of males over 16 years of age had been reported to them in the previous two years. This suggested that the issue had not been taken seriously and is unlikely to represent an accurate picture of the numbers reported.

## Background

It is only recently that assaults on men by men have come under investigation. Little research has therefore been conducted into sexual assaults on men and most of this has relied on samples from medical or social services and is predominantly quantitative. Nielsen (1983) reports that up to 1980 the pronoun 'she' was used almost exclusively in research on sexual abuse survivors. Most of the research until recently has been small in scale (usually about twenty-five men) and predominantly qualitative. The largest epidemiological study ever of unwanted sex on adult males is at present being conducted at the Royal Free Hospital School of Medicine by Michael King and his co-researchers. Preliminary findings indicate that 3 per cent of men in England have been made to suffer or commit unwanted sexual acts since the age of 16 (Coxell *et al.* forthcoming). Mezey and King (1992) carried out a small questionnaire study based at the hospital and King (1992) surveyed male rape in institutions where he concluded that the stigma attached to male rape was even greater than for female rape. This appeared to be one reason few of the victims considered reporting to the police to be a serious option. Most homosexual victims were wary of the police, believing that they would be perceived as 'asking for it' and heterosexuals feared that the police would assume that they must be gay.

Research on the coercive buggery of men indicates that, like the rape of women, sexual violence is more about power and domination than eroticism, as commonly understood. It is the use of sexuality to dominate, humiliate and degrade. The similarities in motive between male and female rape were stressed in the House of Commons during the passage of the Criminal Justice and Public Order Act 1994 (see Rumney and Morgan-Taylor 1997: 26). A common myth is to assume that, because of the nature of the act, male rape is perpetrated by *homosexuals* or seen as a *gay crime*. This is a myth that needs to be dispelled. Paradoxically male rape appears to have more to do with enhancing heterosexuality than to the spread of homosexuality. Research both in the USA and Britain, indicates that male victims are

not chosen for homosexual gratification, but for their apparent vulnerability to violence, so that even infants and old men may be targeted
(McMullen 1990: 24). American studies of rape in prison have shown
that men who are heterosexual will rape men in prison (see Groth
1979). Male prostitutes and homeless men are also vulnerable.

Male rape can therefore be carried out by men who see themselves
in terms of their sexual orientation as predominantly *heterosexual* (see
also Seabrook 1990). McMullen (1990) who set up the first Survivors
group which provides help to victims, argued that male rape is generally carried out by straight men who rape men *they regard as
homosexuals*. The sexual identity of the rapist is then wrongly thought
to be homosexual and homosexuals are blamed for the rape.
McMullen argues that it is very rare for homosexuals to rape.
Although our survey found that gay men did rape other gay men,
overall assailants were more likely to be heterosexual than homosexual. More recent studies have suggested that about half the
perpetrators see themselves as heterosexual. The Survivors help line
stated that of the calls they received in 1991 46 per cent claimed they
were gay, whilst 44 per cent stated they were heterosexual.

## Male rape and the law

It is only recently that non-consensual buggery (anal penetration) has
become incorporated into the rape legislation, a development which
has raised some controversy among feminists who have pointed out
that the change discourages an analysis of the law in gender specific
terms (see Naffine 1994). The Criminal Justice and Public Order Act
1994 (which came into force in January 1995) widened the definition of
rape to include non-consensual penetration of the anus as well as of
the vagina. It carries a maximum sentence of life imprisonment.
Previously such attacks on men had been categorized under indecent
assault, which carried a maximum sentence of ten years' imprisonment
(Section 12, Sexual Offences Act 1956), and buggery of women had
been a criminal offence in itself, whether consensual or not. This
meant that consensual anal sex between heterosexuals was legalized for
the first time. In June 1995 a historical breakthrough was made
following the first conviction for male rape under the new law.[2]

These changes are in line with other countries. Male rape was recognized in New South Wales, Australia in 1981, Sweden in 1984, and
more recently in Germany, Canada, Holland and most US States
(where rape is defined more broadly as non-consensual penetration of
vagina or anus by a penis, hand or other object). The change in the law

followed on from various campaigns by male rape survivors' groups. In New South Wales, Australia the change in the law led to male sexual assault being recognized as a serious health and legal issue, with several sexual assault centres receiving funding for counsellors to work with male clients.[3]

Rendering rape a non-gendered crime raises problems for the feminist explanation of rape as a form of coercion used to keep women subordinate. According to Florence Rush (1990: 170): 'Gender neutrality is rooted in the idea that both genders, male and female, are equally oppressed and that any attempt to hold men and male institutions accountable for transgressions against women is no longer fashionable or acceptable'. Other feminists have expressed concern that men raping men will be seen to be a more serious problem than rape of women and that the male member has been demoted in significance (for a discussion of this see Rumney and Morgan-Taylor 1997: 205–18). However, to include non-consensual buggery of men under the same legislation is not, in our view, to deny the relation between rape, whether of men or women, and male domination, and in particular, domination of the particular hegemonic form of macho masculinity characteristic of Western cultures.

The gender neutrality of the new rape law also raises the question of whether other forms of sexual coercion such as oral sex or penetration with an object should be included in the definition of rape. The definition of buggery has not always been confined to anal penetration as is the case to-day. Weeks (1977: 14) in tracing the development of harsh laws against homosexuality at the close of the nineteenth century points out that 'sodomy was a portmanteau term for any forms of sex that did not have conception as their aim, from homosexual acts to birth control' .

*Prevalence of male rape*

The lack of legal recognition of male rape has meant that few statistics as to its prevalence are available which has contributed to disbelief that it is a problem. According to Gillespie (1996: 152) Home Office figures for 1984–9 indicate that offences of buggery increased by 90 per cent and indecent assault of boys by 24 per cent in England and Wales. The number of men proceeded against for indecent assault of men over 16 years at magistrates' court in 1994 (before the definition of rape was widened to include rape of men) was 532. Of these, 419 were found guilty, an incredibly high rate of conviction. Only 21 of these were dealt with by the Crown Court (Home Office Statistics Division, 2 July

1996). This indicates that comparatively low sentences would have been awarded at the magistrates' courts.

According to the Home Office 1996 statistics, approximately 150 victims of male rape were reported in 1995 (Home Office Statistical Bulletin 1995) the first year the law came into effect. Of those convicted, there were only 2 cases of rape and 2 cases of attempted rape of a male aged 16 and over, and 2 cases of rape and 3 cases of attempted rape of a male aged under 16. Indecent assaults are divided into assaults on boys over 16, those under 16 and buggery by a man with a male person of the age of 16 or over without consent. The numbers of rapes and attempted rapes increased to 227 in 1996, an increase of 51.3 per cent. Compared to over 5,000 reported rapes of women, this is a tiny number but some argue that in certain settings such as prison, a higher proportion of men may be raped than women. Some groups such as male prostitutes may also be particularly at risk (Rumney and Morgan-Taylor 1997: 205).

The number of indecent assaults of male persons 16 years of age or over was 419 and the number of cases of buggery by a man with a male person aged 16 or over without consent was 23. This indicates that the number of rapes on men which reach court are tiny at present. Male rape or non-consensual buggery of men by men is probably one of the most underreported serious crimes in Britain. Only a minority of such assaults are reported to the police. For this reason we know very little about what victims suffer or about the men who carry out the attacks.

It is frequently argued that male rape is even less likely to be reported than female rape. It is impossible to estimate the incidence of such attacks. Some consider that men would be even less likely to report than women, but such comparisons, in our view, are not helpful as we have little clear idea of non-reporting among women. However, men may have even more difficulty than women in talking about such personal issues. As well as the shame that women experience, men's greater unwillingness to admit or talk about their fears relating to criminal victimization is 'a product of men's hesitation to disclose vulnerability' (Stanko and Hobdell 1993: 400). Another important reason why both men and women do not report rape is that they do not think they will be believed. The survey of victims revealed that male complainants were particularly anxious if they had not resisted, which they feared would lead people to assume they had colluded. It can be said that like female rape, the numbers of reported attacks on men has increased over the past decade and overall, a higher number are reaching court.

## The police survey

The police have been urged to adopt a more sympathetic approach to the treatment of rape victims, both male and female, in recent years, and some effort is being made to provide a more user-friendly service. In the early 1990s the Metropolitan Police (the Met.) introduced special training and extended services provided for female victims to male victims. By 1992 the Metropolitan Police had set up a pilot Male Sexual Abuse project and extended the training offered to officers on female rape to male rape, training 26 officers to act as 'chaperones' to take statements from victims and remain attached to the cases until the investigation had been completed. This meant taking them off other duties. All chaperones must have completed the Sexual Offences Investigative Techniques Course. It is emphasized that all victims, regardless of sex or race will be treated with kindness, sensitivity and courtesy by all employees of the Met. All chaperones must be conversant with the CPS booklet 'Advice for Victims of Sexual Assault'. A male or female officer, depending on the wishes of the victim, will wherever possible be appointed as chaperone by a detective inspector. According to the guidelines for investigators, chaperones should not be employed in this role more than two or three times a year. Chaperones have two crucial functions. First, to ensure that victims are treated with kindness, sensitivity and courtesy, and second, to obtain the best possible evidence to aid an investigation and support any subsequent prosecution.

The police guidelines for investigators and chaperones states that whenever doubts arise investigating officers must bear the following two principles in mind:

- The interests of the victim and the victim's wishes may only be overridden in exceptional circumstances.
- It is policy of the Met. to accept as the truth all aspects of an allegation made by any victim. An allegation will only be considered as falling short of a substantiated allegation after a full enquiry.

Treatment for serious sexual physical injuries should be given in hospital before the forensic examination; forensic examinations should be undertaken in a rape suite by a doctor of the victim's preference; the victim's account should be believed unless there is strong contradictory evidence and even if the allegation is withdrawn, a full investigation should occur. Such schemes have spread across the country in the last five years.

## Results of the survey

Analysis of both police and victim questionnaires shows that police officers are more likely to regard the testimony of homosexual victims as 'unreliable' – i.e. either to assume that the sex was consensual or that the complainant was malicious. Feedback from gay victims suggests that this scepticism is unfounded. Indeed gay victims are less likely to report, so false allegations are most unlikely to occur.

Victim feedback also indicated that gay men are treated less sensitively and sympathetically by the police than heterosexual men. Some police officers seem to believe that rape is less traumatic for gay men.

At the time of this survey less that half (43 per cent) of interviewing officers had had special training in dealing with victims of male rape. In the Metropolitan Police the average was 57 per cent of 213 completed questionnaires. Three forces – Northumbria, Sussex and Leicestershire – had introduced training for all interviewing officers, but only one completed questionnaire was returned. This suggests that there is great variability throughout the country both in relation to the availability of training and the recognition of the offence.

When interviewed by researchers, police officers expressed feelings of inadequacy in dealing with these offences and many felt ill-equipped to deal sensitively with the victims. Officers with many years of CID experience reported that they had never encountered a report of this type. They wanted more information, guidance and training and regretted that little was known about male rape – both in terms of offending behaviour and the effects on the victims.

A total of 50 (83 per cent) of the reported rapes involved single assailants; 10 (17 per cent) involved more than one assailant. Roughly the same number of reported rapes involved strangers (21 or 35 per cent) as involved assailants whom the victim had known for longer than 24 hours (22 or 37 per cent). Only 13 (22 per cent) had met within 24 hours and 2 (7 per cent) involved co-prisoners or cellmates in prison. As with female rape, the majority (two-thirds) of male rapes are by suspects who are acquainted with their victims in some way. In other words sudden violent assaults by strangers are relatively rare. Most male rapists will use a 'conning' approach or exploit the fact that they are in a position of trust to gain control over the victim. The location in which the assaults took place is similar to equivalent data for female rape and reflects the fact that most victims have some previous acquaintance with the suspect. The majority of rapes (55 per cent) take place indoors – either in the victim's home (19 per cent) or the suspect's home (36 per cent).

Two-thirds of the victims reported to the police on the same day or the day after the incident. Almost half, 27 (47 per cent) reported the same day. However, one in ten men took several days to report and 18 per cent took several weeks, months or years before reporting. The proportion of women reporting after a delay may be even higher although nationwide figures are not available. In the evaluation report of REACH (Rape Examination, Advice, Counselling and Help) conducted by Maddock and Scott (1995) 27 per cent of female rape victims made their first contact more than twelve months after the assault.

Analysis of police questionnaires showed that the majority of assailants make some attempt to 'arouse' male victims through fellatio or masturbation; 56 per cent involved other sexual acts, most commonly forced fellatio performed on the victim (46 per cent). This can be just as distressing for the victim as the act of buggery. Additionally over a quarter (28 per cent) of the assailants forced the victim to perform sexual acts on them – e.g. most commonly fellatio but also masturbation. In three cases, the assailant forced the victim to reciprocate and anally penetrate them also.

Forcing men to take part in what is regarded as homosexual acts, often leads victims to be confused about their own sexual orientation. Victims sometimes have erections and even ejaculate which can undermine their feelings of self worth as they feel that in some way they are colluding with their assailant (McMullen 1990: 73). Fear that they will be considered to be homosexual also leads many to have qualms about reporting to the police. Research has shown that victims sometimes assume that the perpetrator was gay and thus they must be giving off gay signals which incited the act (Mezey and King 1992). For men who are gay, the barriers to reporting may be even greater as they may assume that the police are homophobic. According to Ford Hickson at the University of Portsmouth, who set up Project Sigma, an investigatory study into 1,000 men who identified themselves as gay, gay men tend not to report to the police as they think it would be harder for them to prove lack of consent in view of the myths regarding the promiscuity of gay men.

Such myths need to be challenged. It is important that police officers understand that penile erections need have nothing to do with pleasure. Kinsey (1948), the American psychologist who carried out the first survey of the incidence of homosexual behaviour in the United States, found that erections could arise from non-sexual stimulation. In his investigation into adolescent boys who had been sexually assaulted by men, he discovered that violence and non-erotic stimuli and horseplay can lead to erection and even to ejaculation. He published a list of emotional states in which boys experience sexual excitation including erection, and ejaculation. The list includes among others, being scared, fearing punishment, anger, and being yelled at. Kinsey (1948: 164–5) concludes 'the record suggests that the physiological mechanism of any emotional response (anger, fright, pain etc.) may be the mechanism of sexual response. These reactions need have nothing to do with sexual desire or pleasure'. The act of anal penetration stimulates the prostate gland and an erection in such cases is automatic. Apparently stimulation of the prostate gland can cause an automatic erection in impotent and disabled men. According to King's epidemiological study (1992) 20 per cent of men assaulted by men got an erection or ejaculated.

Male rape may precipitate a crisis of sexual identity. As Adler (1992: 128) points out:

> when the victim is male, any claim that he consented projects on to him a homosexual identity....Where the victim is heterosexual, the very fear of being thought a homosexual may well stop him from reporting. In fact, the reasons for not reporting for male victims are much the same as they are for female victims, and include shock, embarrassment, fear, self blame and a high degree of stigma.

They may question their masculinity and doubt their manhood. According to McMullen (1990) who set up Survivors, a helpline for men, it is not unusual for heterosexual victims to actively seek homosexual contacts after having been raped.

### Characteristics of assaults

The majority of the rapes reported to the police involved indecent sexual acts other than anal penetration. As we have seen, almost half of the men had forced fellatio on the victim. In three cases the assailant forced the victim to reciprocate by penetrating them. Several gay victims commented that a common misconception is that all gay men practise anal sex. This is by no means the case. Police officers interviewing gay victims should be aware that anal sex has a particular significance in the gay community. It is seldom carried out in 'casual' relationships but almost always between partners in long-term relationships of love and trust. This is partly because anal sex can be extremely painful if the person penetrated is not relaxed and also, because of the fear of HIV, the person penetrating must be trusted to wear a condom. Indeed it is because anal penetration is most commonly an act of intimacy and love between gay men, that rape is just as great a violation for gay men as for heterosexual men. One man interviewed by the TV researchers described his sexual orientation as gay but in regard to the assault commented that: 'this was the first time I had been penetrated'.

Male victims of rape are just as unlikely to resist the attack – either physically or verbally – as female rape victims, irrespective of their age or physical build. Only around a third of male victims offer any resistance to their assailants. Despite the common misconception that men ought to be able to fight back, victims should be reassured that to resist is fairly uncommon. The amount of physical or verbal resistance by victims was not related to the amount of violence actually used or threatened. A total of 60 per cent (36) offered no resistance, and only 17 per cent (10) physically resisted. A further 23 per cent (14) offered verbal resistance.

The police survey showed that extreme violence is not usually necessary to carry out rapes on men (see Table 5.1). Weapons were used in less than a quarter of cases, and weapons combined with physical violence (like punching and kicking) used in less than half the cases. The threat of violence was usually sufficient to gain compliance. There were no major differences in the degree of violence used in stranger and acquaintance rapes. Stranger rapists were more likely to use weapons (for example, knives were used in 28 per cent of cases compared to 17 per cent in the acquaintance group) but the latter were more likely to use threats to kill. On analysis actual injuries sustained tended to be greater in the acquaintance group.

These findings indicate that police officers should be sensitive to the diversity of sexual acts that take place during assaults and particularly to the likelihood that the assailant will have forced or attempted to force the victim to perform sexual acts on them. If the victim complied, and most are too afraid not to, they most commonly suffer great shame and guilt. It is therefore important that police officers are able to reassure the victim that this is a common feature of male rapes and that they are by no means unusual.

### Gang rapes

Assailants in gang rape were more likely to be young and were more likely to be black than in single rapes. Altogether there were ten gang rapes, seven of which involved defendants who were complete

*Table 5.1* Incidence of violence

| | | |
|---|---|---|
| Forcibly held down | 20 | 37% |
| Tied or handcuffed | 2 | 4% |
| Punched, kicked, strangled | 12 | 12% |
| Weapon used | 12 | 22% |
| Weapon threatened | 6 | 11% |
| Threat to kill | 12 | 22% |
| Non-specific threat | 5 | 9% |
| Threat to harm | 1 | 2% |
| Given drugs | 2 | 4% |
| Blackmail | 2 | 4% |

*Notes*:
Number of cases where the extent of violence used was known totals 54
Percentages add up to more than 100 due to assailants using more than one type of violence to control the victim.

strangers. In regard to the ages of the assailants, in six cases the ages were known and in five of these the men involved were between 22 and 30 years of age. Three of these seven stranger gang rapes involved at least one black assailant. One involved three, another two and the third involved one black suspect (who was accompanied by a white suspect). Since all the victims of these rapes were white Europeans it is possible that these rapes could have had a racial motive. More research is needed to investigate such rapes.

In regard to sexual orientation, four of the victims were described as homosexual, three as heterosexual, one as bisexual and in two cases the sexuality of the victim was unknown. Given that the majority of victims overall were heterosexual, this data suggests that homosexual men may be more vulnerable to attacks by gang rapists which in many cases may be homophobic attacks.

## Characteristics of victims and suspects

Police officers were asked to indicate what they believed the sexual orientation of suspects to be. Out of 72 assailants, they classified only 9 (13 per cent) as heterosexual, 21 (29 per cent) as homosexual, 13 (18 per cent) as bisexual and 29 (40 per cent) as not known.

These figures indicate that the police assume that most attackers must be bisexual if they know them to have heterosexual relationships. There appears to be a strong tendency for the police to see male rape as a predominantly homosexual crime.

Information on the sexual orientation of suspects is clearly much more reliable in cases where the victim had known the suspect for more than 24 hours (see Table 5.2). In 12 out of 22 cases (55 per cent of acquaintance male rapes), the suspect was having or had had sexual relationships with women. In 27 per cent of acquaintance rapes one or more of the suspects were married or cohabiting with a female at the time of the offence. These findings suggest that most suspects are either heterosexual or pursue heterosexual lifestyles. The data also suggests that heterosexual or bisexual suspects are more likely to attack men who are heterosexual than homosexual.

Only two homosexual victims reported acquaintance rape to the police which confirms that gay men are much less likely to report this type of rape.

Out of 50 cases where the ages of the victims were specified, 17 (34 per cent) were aged between 16 to 20 years, 11 (22 per cent) were described as educationally subnormal (ESN) and no ages specified, and 10 (20 per cent) were aged 21 to 25. Clearly young men were the most likely targets of male rapists, probably due to their vulnerability. The large number of victims described as ESN is also a matter of concern.

Over half (26, or 52 per cent) the suspects were over the age of 30. This group of men were most likely to attack victims under 21 or those who are educationally subnormal. Less than a quarter of their victims were of a similar age to themselves. Fifteen (or 30 per cent) were aged 22–30 years. Younger suspects were more likely to attack men of roughly their own age group or older. Only 13 per cent of their victims were under 21 or ESN.

This is a very different profile from assailants who attack women, where the majority are under 25 (Brownmiller 1978: 176, Lees 1997a: 227). It is possible that the greater number of older assailants in this

Table 5.2 Assumed sexual orientation of suspects and victims

|  | Hetero-sexual victim | Homo-sexual victim | Bisexual victim | Victim's orientation not known | Total suspects |
|---|---|---|---|---|---|
| Heterosexual suspect | 3 | 0 | 0 | 2 | 5 |
| Homosexual suspect | 1 | 1 | 1 | 3 | 6 |
| Bisexual suspect | 4 | 1 | 0 | 2 | 7 |
| Not known | 1 | 0 | 0 | 3 | 4 |

*Note*:
Cases where victim/suspect were known to each other longer than 24 hours total 22.

sample is due to the limited access older men have to younger women as opposed to younger men. This assumes that some rapists may progress from raping young women to raping young men.

### Previous criminal record

In 19 of the cases of reported rape, information on the previous criminal record of the assailants was not available, usually because no suspect was identified or interviewed. The majority of 'unknown' cases were stranger rapes. In 41 cases information was available (see Table 5.3). The vast majority of the 'known' cases were rapes by acquaintances. Since two suspects were charged with two rapes, the total number of suspects for whom information was available was 39. The vast majority of suspects (29 or 74 per cent) had previous criminal convictions and half the suspects (19 or 49 per cent) had been given a prison sentence for past criminal activities. Only 10 (26 per cent) had no previous record. The most common conviction was for some kind of dishonesty, such as burglary. Most suspects (58 per cent) with a prior criminal record were 'generalists' – i.e. they had previously committed more than one type of offence.

The majority had no record of sex offences. However, 10 men had previous convictions for sexual offences against men and two of these it should be noted, had a previous conviction for sex offences against females. In almost two thirds of cases, the suspect's prior criminal activity was serious enough to warrant a prison sentence. Those who had previous convictions for sexual offences were also likely to have convictions for other types of offences on their record, most commonly offences involving dishonesty.

*Table 5.3* Breakdown of previous crimes committed by suspects in male rape cases

|  | No. of suspects | % total suspects (39) | % suspects with criminal record (29) |
|---|---|---|---|
| No previous convictions | 10 | 26 | — |
| Sex offences against males | 10 | 26 | 35 |
| Sex offences against females | 2 | 5 | 7 |
| Violent offences | 13 | 33 | 45 |
| Dishonesty offences | 22 | 56 | 76 |
| Prior prison/young offenders institution sentence | 19 | 49 | 66 |

## Identification and disposal of suspects

A suspect or suspects were identified in 45 out of 60 cases of male rape, giving an overall identification rate of 75 per cent. However, in 38 of the 45 cases, the victim was able to name the suspect. When identification rates were analysed on the basis of the relationships to the victim, the results were as follows:

| | |
|---|---|
| Victim knew suspect longer than 24 hours | 100 per cent named suspect |
| Victim knew suspect less than 24 hours | 94 per cent named suspect |
| Stranger | 22 per cent named suspect |

A suspect or suspects were interviewed in 40 out of the 60 cases of male rape. It is likely that some of these cases may have been 'no crimed', whereas in others an arrest may have been made. Unfortunately we do not have this information. Regarding 'no criming', according to the Met. policy guidelines for investigators:

> unless the allegation is classified as 'no crime' beforehand, any suspect named or later identified must be interviewed. The only exception to this rule may be where, despite having named a suspect, the victim asks police not to approach the suspect for fear of reprisal or because they do not want to support a prosecution. Authority not to interview a suspect in these circumstances must be obtained from the area detective chief superintendent. While it will sometimes be appropriate to interview the alleged offender and take forensic samples, it could be difficult to justify placing the victim at further risk by alerting the suspect to the fact that the case has been reported to the police. The detective superintendent should weigh up the interests of the victim against what is known about the current patterns of criminal activity, with particular attention to linked or series offences. It may be that the needs of the victim will have to take second place to the greater needs of the public good. However, the first principle dictates that a decision to interview against the victim's wishes should be rare.

In 5 cases, all where the victim knew the suspect well, no interview took place. In 4 cases this decision was taken by the police and, in one case, on the advice of the Crown Prosecution Service. The reasons given in two cases by the police for not interviewing the suspect were that the complainant had withdrawn the allegations, and in the remaining cases the complainants were considered unreliable witnesses. In one of these cases the unreliable complainant was a 21-year-old male prostitute. The police officer commented: 'He is described by his friends as very promiscuous'. This is not a good reason for failing to interview him as male prostitutes are very unlikely to report acts of consensual sex to the police. In another case, the complainant was a 25-year-old homosexual who had answered an advertisement in a gay magazine, and the questionnaire mentioned the possibility of the man being mentally ill. The decision not to investigate is unfortunate given the feasibility that some male rapists might specifically 'target' vulnerable victims through contact magazines.

A suspect or suspects were charged in only 22 out of 60 (37 per cent) of cases. In other words, there were a further 18 cases where suspects were interviewed, but not charged. In 8 cases the decision not to charge the suspect was taken by the police, and in 9 cases by the CPS (see Table 5.4). In one case the suspect escaped while on bail before he could be charged.

In the cases where the decision not to charge the suspect was taken by the police the reasons were as follows: in 5 cases there was insufficient evidence, and in 3 cases the victim was unwilling to give evidence. The issue of victims' unwillingness to give evidence has been discussed above.

Where suspects were interviewed but the cases were dropped, in 3 cases it does not appear that there was sufficient evidence that the right suspect had been caught. In 2 further cases both complainants were described by the police as educationally subnormal. In one of these cases, of a 19-year-old allegedly raped by a friend, there was forensic evidence in the form of sperm round the anus. In the second case, another 19-year-old allegedly raped by an acquaintance had internal bleeding in the anus, and the suspect had previous convictions for violent offences, and had served a prison sentence. In addition, police

*Table 5.4* Reasons given by CPS not to prosecute

| | |
|---|---|
| Issue of consent: | 3 |
| Insufficient evidence | 5 |
| Trauma for complainant of giving evidence in court | 1 |
| Total | 9 |

had information on their files about a similar allegation for which the suspect had not been prosecuted. It appears to indicate that the police are not prepared to take cases forward where the complainants are ESN.

In one case involving an alleged stranger attack, the complainant was a 44-year-old heterosexual male. The reasons were not given for why he was considered unreliable, but the officer did comment that the complainant, when interviewed, said he had been sexually assaulted many times before. While the complainant may have been lying on this occasion, his description of what happened during the assault was typical of genuine rapes, and, there was forensic evidence that sex had taken place (i.e. cuts and bruises around the anus). In any event such allegations should be taken seriously unless there is clear evidence that the complainant is lying.

The stigma of male rape is such that many complainants are still not likely to proceed with a prosecution unless given great emotional support by the police, particularly in cases where they know the assailant. Assailants also place pressure on the victim not to proceed. If the police or the CPS decide not to prosecute, the evidence will still be kept for use in any future prosecution of the same suspect in relation to other victims. In cases which are 'no crimed' or unsolved, a report must be sent within three months to the area operational command unit senior detective superintendent for authority to close the investigation and put the papers away.

Regarding the issue of consent, in one case the 17-year-old complainant was described as a 'rent boy'. In this case the suspect had previous convictions for sex offences against males and had served time in prison. In the two other cases, both (heterosexual) 19-year-old complainants had been allegedly raped by other inmates in prison.

While it is likely that 'rent boys' and criminals are less likely to be believed by a jury than complainants of good character, it is nevertheless difficult to justify the decision of the CPS not to press charges in these cases, rather than allow a jury to decide on the issue of consent.

Regarding the grounds of insufficient evidence, all 5 cases where the CPS decided that there was insufficient evidence to prosecute involved suspects known to the victim (for longer than 24 hours). In 3 of the 5 cases, the victims were described by police as ESN. In all 3 cases, the CPS were concerned about the complainants' ability to give reliable evidence and cope with cross-examination in court. Two cases involved the same suspect – a social worker who worked with the clients with 'special educational needs'. He had no previous convictions. In the third case, the suspect was over 50 and retired with no previous convictions. In the fourth case, that of a 17 year old, the complainant may also have had special needs. The police officer commented that the CPS 'thought the victim would be unable to cope well with cross-examination'. The suspect in this case had previous convictions for sex offences against males, violence and dishonesty and had served time in prison.

In the final case, involving several offences against an 18-year-old male over a three year period, it is also unclear why the CPS took the decision not to prosecute. However, once again the victim may have been considered 'too vulnerable' by the CPS to give evidence in court. In this case the suspect was described as a 'hostel warden' with no previous convictions, but with one previous unsubstantiated allegation of a similar nature by a different complainant.

In the case where the CPS decided not to press charges on the grounds that it would be too traumatic for the complainant, according to the police officer, the complainant had 'moderate learning difficulties' and the CPS believed that 'in court no account would be taken by the defence of his difficulties'. Sexual assaults on men with learning difficulties is an unresearched area but recent research on such women indicates that it may well be widespread in institutions (McCarthy 1996) and few such cases result in a Crown Court hearing.

Suspects were prosecuted in only 4 such cases. In one of these the defendant was charged on three indictments of non-consensual buggery. He pleaded guilty to three counts of indecent assault and received a mere fifteen month sentence of imprisonment. In the two other cases that reached court, both defendants pleaded not guilty. In both cases the judge directed an acquittal on the grounds that the complainants were unable to give reliable evidence on account of their educational difficulties. Of additional concern is the fact that both defendants had previous criminal convictions for sex offences against males. The police survey suggests that those who rape ESN victims can do so with impunity.

None of the ten gang rapes led to successful prosecutions. Seven of

*Table 5.5* Prosecution rates according to the relationship to the victim

| | |
|---|---|
| 10 out of 16 of the general acquaintance group were prosecuted | 63% |
| 9 out of 26 of the intimate group were prosecuted | 35% |
| 2 out of 18 of the stranger group were prosecuted | 11% |

the ten were by complete strangers. Six were sudden attacks in an outdoor area such as a park. In the seventh case, the assailants conned their way into the victim's home. In none of the seven cases of gang rape by strangers was a suspect identified or interviewed.

Three of the ten gang rapes were 'acquaintance' rapes – i.e. involving at least one suspect previously known to the victim. Although suspects were identified in all three cases, in only one case was a suspect interviewed. In all three acquaintance cases, the victims later withdrew their allegations and no further actions was taken by the police. It is possible that two of the acquaintance 'gang' rapes may have been connected. Both took place in the Met. area and one of the men involved in each case was aged 46 to 50 years, an unusual age for gang rapists. This suspect was interviewed in connection with one of the rapes and is described as having previous criminal convictions which include sexual offences against males and females, as well as prior convictions for violence and dishonesty offences.

Twenty-three per cent (14 out of 60) of the total police sample were deemed to be ESN. This suggests that these types of complainants are vulnerable to attacks by male rapists, or are more likely to report to the police. It does appear to be iniquitous that in the vast majority of such cases, no suspect was prosecuted although, in 13 out of 14 of these cases, a suspect was named by the complainant. Suspects were prose- cuted in only 4 such cases. One case was awaiting committal at the time the data was collected. In one case the defendant was charged on three indictments of non-consensual buggery. He pleaded guilty to three counts of indecent assault and was given a fifteen month sentence.

Regarding the two other cases that reached court, both defendants pleaded not guilty. In both cases, the judge directed an acquittal on the grounds that the complainants were unable to give reliable evidence. This was in spite of the defendant's past criminal record which included convictions for sex offences against males.

Twenty out of sixty cases were committed for trial. Ten cases were still awaiting a hearing and in one case the suspect committed suicide before the trial. Of the nine cases which did reach Crown Court, 81 per cent resulted in a successful conviction. When these nine cases are analyzed on the basis of the relationship to the victim the results are as shown in Table 5.6.

These figures are very small so it is dangerous to drawn any firm conclusions from them. It is worth noting, however, that although the proportion of cases reaching Crown Court is relatively low (20 out of 60), this is still considerably higher than the proportion of cases of

*Table 5.6* Numbers of convictions according to relationship with victim

| | | |
|---|---|---|
| Those acquainted for over 24 hours | 3 out of 4 prosecutions successful | 75% |
| Those acquainted less than 24 hours | 4 out of 5 prosecutions successful | 80% |
| Stranger | 2 out of 2 prosecutions successful | 100% |

rape of females reaching Crown Court (1 in 3 compared to 1 in 4). These figures also suggest that juries may be more willing to convict in cases where the victim is male. Home Office statistics on female rape show that only one in four cases reach court of which about 30 per cent result in a conviction (Home Office Statistics 1996) compared with the above figures of between 75 and 100 per cent.

Although male rape is now illegal, very few cases reach the Crown Court. There is also evidence that judges are still not aware that male erections can be caused by fear and induced by coercion rather than through consent. In a case heard in April 1995, the victim, a young heterosexual man who had been raped while on remand in prison by a 40-year-old man who was coming to the end of serving a ten year sentence, was questioned about the fact that he had had an erection and the following cross-examination ensued:

DEFENCE COUNSEL:  Nothing in your behaviour would have indicated that you were not consenting – yes?
VICTIM:  Just lying there is giving consent, is it? Getting a hard on is giving consent? Does it actually: yes, bum me – please do it now?...I feel if a person is to give consent, they give consent through their mouth'.

(Official court transcript)

The judge stopped the case on the grounds that this was evidence of consent and did not even allow the jury to consider the matter. It is most unlikely that the situation has improved since then which indicates that there is a vital need for training to be introduced for the judges and the CPS.

Prison sentences were known for seven of those convicted and ranged from eighteen months (where the offender had no previous convictions) to fourteen years. The average sentence was six years.

## Making sense of male rape

### Reinforcing hegemonic masculinity

Enforcing and maintaining the dominant (or hegemonic) form of masculinity is not only achieved through violence towards women but violence towards other subordinated and marginalized groups. Connell (1987) is one of the first contemporary sociologists to analyse the relation between power and masculinity. He challenged the assumption that masculinity is a unitary construct and pointed out the diversity of masculinities. Of particular significance to the understanding of male rape was the importance of analysing the relations between these different kinds of masculinity; relations of alliance, dominance and subordination. These relationships are constructed through various practices or systems of representation within certain social contexts such as the school, the workplace and sport. Such practices exclude and include, and involve power relations between different groups of men. Connell refers to the dominant form as *hegemonic*, by which he suggests the exercise of power through moral authority underpinned by the threat of violence (see Kenway 1995). Men raping men and men raping women can both be seen as forms of promoting dominant hegemonic heterosexuality.

There are all kinds of all-male activities – from initiation ceremonies of the Masons, to football 'hooliganism' and drinking binges – which can be seen to enhance male solidarity. Connell (1995: 31) describes how in some societies various kinds of homosexual behaviour have been regarded as central to the survival of the society. He describes the initiation rituals of the 'guardians of the flutes' in the highlands of Papua New Guinea which involved the sustained sexual relations between boy initiates and young adult men in which the penis is sucked and semen swallowed. The semen is regarded as the essence of masculinity that must be transmitted between generations of men to ensure the survival of society.

Likewise, Walker (1988), who undertook a study of the relations between boys in school in Australia, shows how hegemonic forms of masculinity among boys leads to derogating everything feminine or related to femininity in order to purge masculine identity from any such association. This wards off threats to gender identity and 'reduce(s) the level of disgust and revulsion caused by "poofs" and any undermining of male authority by females who were less submissive than it was thought they should be' (Benson and Walker 1988: 90). In the US, as reported by Connell (1995: 218–19), the early 1990s have seen a new wave of homophobic campaigns depicting gay men as 'an army of lawbreakers, violating God's commands, threatening first the family and then the larger social order'.

### Understanding homophobia

The homophobia evident in Walker's (1988) ethnographic study of Australian school culture is evident in educational studies carried out in this country. Beynon's (1989) study of a tough English secondary school is a good example. Beynon sees violence at the heart of contemporary masculinity which must be understood in the context of social structures, relationships and interactions. Encoded messages regarding masculinity, and by implication femininity, were embedded in all kinds of social practices. Violence took different forms in the day to day life of the school he studied and was not merely condoned but sanctioned by the ethos of the school. Some teachers physically assaulted boys, who were hit, pushed and shaken. He found that in the lower school a hard core of male teachers regarded coercive measures as synonymous with 'good' teaching and a virtue to be upheld. Teachers were generally prepared to write off most pupil violence as normal, healthy boyish exuberance and horseplay. Much of the violence was homophobic and there were widespread attacks on boys regarded as 'queers' or 'poofs'. The same effeminate boys were often rejected by many teachers.

Homophobia appeared to be the motive in a number of attacks in the findings of the *Dispatches* (1994) documentary on male rape. Raping gays or men who are perceived as 'weaker' can paradoxically be seen as a way of defending oneself against homosexual feelings. When carried out with a friend or gang, rape can be seen as both a way of enhancing relationships with them (victims often report that the assailants laughed and joked with each other) and, by humiliating the victim, of showing oneself to be a 'real man'. Humiliation was reported by many assailants, some of whom had been left lying naked and wounded in the street or urinated on.

The control of consensual sexual relations and homosexual desire between men has always been a particular concern of all male communities, groups or institutions such as the armed forces. The law against homosexuality (buggery) was introduced to control such behaviour in the navy in the nineteenth century. In 1816, for example, four members of the crew of the Royal Africaine were hanged for buggery after a major naval scandal (see Weeks 1983: 13). The death penalty for this crime was re-enacted in 1826 by Sir Robert Peel at the same time it was removed for over a hundred other crimes. It was abandoned in 1836 and finally abolished in 1861. According to Weeks (1983:13) the armed services believed themselves to have special problems of order and discipline since 'sexual contact between men and especially across ranks, threatened to tear asunder the carefully maintained hierarchy'. There is a delicate balance between enhancing male camaraderie at the same time as controlling sexual relations between them which could so easily disrupt the patterns of authority and class. The expression of sexuality as a form of power and humiliation on the other hand, as in male rape, could be used as part of military strategy both as a means of enhancing masculinity within battalions and as a strategy of war. According to some authorities (see Seabrook 1990), non-consensual buggery is a common practice of invading armies where the defeated are raped in order to break their spirit. It is estimated that 10 per cent of the rapes in Bosnia were of defeated men (Stiglmayer 1993).

## Conclusion

This study indicates that some police forces are beginning to take assaults on men seriously, but less than half of interviewing officers had had any special training in dealing with victims. Most cases involved assaults by acquaintances and most assaults involved a variety of sexual acts, some of which the victim was forced to perform on the defendant. Many victims felt very guilty about such participation, so it is important that police officers are aware of this and can reassure victims that their response is perfectly normal for those who are under coercion. It should also be emphasized that male victims are no more likely to resist than female victims, even when they are faced with no extreme violence. One of the most relevant findings for police practice is that as many as half the perpetrators were identified by victims as predominantly heterosexual, although police records indicated that perpetrators tended to be seen as predominantly homosexual or bisexual. All these factors indicate that adequate training is essential if the police are to understand the particular problems involved with male rape and are not to exacerbate the suffering of victims by insensitive or callous treatment.

# 6    Complainants' views of the police

## Background

One of the main aims of our research was to interview complainants to find out their views of police service delivery and other services, such as Victim Support and Rape Crisis. In the next two chapters the findings of this aspect of our research will be reviewed. Chapter 6 outlines the effect of sexual assault on complainants and the response of the police from the time the rape is reported until the case, if it proceeds, is heard in the Crown Court. Chapter 7 reports on the short-comings of the medical examination, the experience women have in court and their assessment of Victim Support and Rape Crisis services. As we explained in Chapter 3, all women who had been sexually assaulted between 1988 and 1990 and had reported the attack to one of the two police stations were contacted. Discussions were held with various police officers including members of the child protection team and a forensic medical examiner.

Contacting women who have been raped is no easy task and we considered several different possibilities. We approached Victim Support, but after several discussions we decided it might be confusing for complainants to be given details of a research project by a coun-selling agency. Since we had gained the co-operation of the police, the best line of action seemed to be to ask them if they would be willing to send out a letter from us. They agreed to do this on condition that we composed a letter for them to send out since it would be a breach of confidentiality to give us the names and addresses of complainants. This meant that we were unable to write to women directly. We also wrote an article for a local newspaper, as a result of which we were able to make contact with two complainants who had been raped in the area and had reported it to the police.

The letter to the complainants explained why we wanted to hear their views and asked if they were willing to be interviewed about the treatment they had received from the police, police surgeons, the court and other agencies. This method carried the risk of associating our research too closely with the police. Two women assumed the letter we had sent out was from the police, although it specifically stated that we were independent researchers. Their confusion is understandable, but unavoidable since the letter was written on police note paper; this may have deterred some women from replying.

Great sensitivity is needed in undertaking this type of research and analyzing the material is disturbing. We made it clear in the letter to respondents that we would not be asking them any details about the rape itself, but wanted to find out about their experiences after reporting the assault. However, in practice it is difficult to make such a clear cut distinction and the very process of remembering what happened at the police station inevitably brings to mind the assault itself. We tried as far as possible to glean information from the records so as to avoid asking questions about the assault itself. As Hanmer *et al.* (1994) have pointed out, there is a possibility that the research process itself can become a form of violence if it is not conducted in a sensitive and /or empowering way. Confidentiality is crucial in this area and we made sure that all the women were aware that we would not use their real names. In some cases we were able to inform women about the outcome of their court case where they had not been told. In several cases women said that it had been helpful talking to us although their main motivation had been to improve the process for other women.

## Treatment of rape complainants

As we have seen in Chapter 1, the police treatment of rape complainants has radically changed since police policy was to let a woman 'make her statement and then drive a coach and horses through it'.[1] In the London area where our research was undertaken, special police officers undergo a week's training at Hendon, the Metropolitan Police training college, before being assigned to sexual assault cases. Additionally, some sixty-four special units to deal with domestic attacks were set up in London, including two in Islington, and a rape examination suite away from the main police stations now operates. We visited this and found it was clean and fairly well equipped but we were a little nonplussed by the difficulty the police had in identifying where the key was kept. It did not appear to be used very often and had a clinical air about it.

We interviewed four detective inspectors who all maintained that the police reaction to the Thames Valley documentary of a woman facing harsh interrogation techniques (see Chapter 1) had had a tremendous impact on the force. They outlined exactly how the procedures now worked. Rule number 1 is, to quote the Metropolitan Police guidelines, that 'it is the policy of the Metropolitan Police Service to accept as the truth all aspects of an allegation made by any victim. An allegation will only be considered as falling short of a substantiated allegation after a full enquiry' (Metropolitan Police 1995: 2). As King and Brown (1997: 1) state, 'at the centre of the Metropolitan Police's philosophy is the acceptance of the truth of all aspects of an allegation made by the victim unless good reasons are evident of fabrication'.

As soon as the woman is fit enough, a female officer takes a statement. This account is then passed to the detective inspector so that he or she knows what they are dealing with. The doctor is called and the woman is then taken to a rape examination suite for examination. The suites are used for cases of serious indecent assault as well as rape. The doctor takes samples of bodily fluids, pubic hair, nail samples etc. in order that DNA information can be obtained for identification purposes. Forensic doctors and victim support workers may be called as witnesses. A crime report form is completed as the first step in the administrative process and the crime is given a number. The crime classification is normally done within seven days, but it can take longer, as we have seen.

This is one of the first studies to interview women who have reported sexual assault since these developments have taken place. Little research into the experiences of women who have been raped has been carried out in Britain. Chambers and Millar (1983) of the Scottish Office Central Research Unit, as we saw in Chapter 1, interviewed 70 women who had been sexually assaulted, 40 of whom were victims of rape. Views expressed by complainants about CID officers and WPCs were mainly negative and critical. In the main the criticisms were concentrated on the unsympathetic and tactless manner in which interviewing was often conducted. Just under 50 per cent considered the police had done a good job of the investigation, and, overall, they concluded that there was general dissatisfaction. Chambers and Millar (1983) argued that the main reason for this was that there was widespread belief that complaints of rape were often false. This is in spite of the lack of evidence that fabricated allegations of rape occur more than in other crimes (see Temkin 1987). However, individual officers found it very difficult to document individual cases that fitted into the category of false complaints. Another study was undertaken by

Adler in 1991. Rather than interviewing women, she carried out a postal survey to which 103 women who had reported rape and whose offences had been 'crimed' by the police between May 1990 and February 1991 responded. The women indicated in the questionnaires that they were generally satisfied with the way they had been treated by the police. One woman, however, was critical of the way she was questioned and had been told 'to expect far worse in court' (Adler 1991: 1115).

Two other important developments have influenced the way rape is handled. Firstly, during the 1980s research has advanced our knowledge about the short- and long-term effects of rape – often referred to as the rape trauma syndrome, a post-traumatic stress response (see Holmstrom and Burgess 1978, Hall 1985, Mezey and Taylor 1988, Newburn 1993). Typical reactions include helplessness (see Williams and Holmes 1981), sleeplessness, flashbacks, nightmares, anger, suicidal feelings, phobic reactions, depression, mood swings, fear of being alone, relationship problems (in particular not enjoying sex), anorexia, loss of concentration and self-esteem and blaming oneself. Personal relationships are disrupted, and sexual relationships often break up. A finding of crucial importance is that such reactions are frequently delayed. In other words the experiences are 'blocked out'. Therefore, complainants may often appear calm and controlled, or they may be angry rather than distraught. These are common responses to other traumas too. Forensic doctors need to be aware of such reactions and be careful what implications they draw from the complainant's demeanour, as these can be very prejudicial in court as we shall see in Chapter 7.

The use of a medical term, rape trauma syndrome, to describe such symptoms has some disadvantages. Absence of particular symptoms can be used maliciously by defence doctors for example, as evidence that the complainant is making false allegations or has not been raped. One of the ironies is that the very qualities that help women survive are the ones that are most inappropriate for obtaining a conviction; the rape victim is expected to display emotion even many months after the event and in public. The use of medical terms can also reduce the complexity of the woman's experiences to a set of 'individual symptoms' which once understood can be cured by the medical profession alone (see Foley 1994: 44). It can also give the impression that the reactions are psychopathological rather than normal. On the other hand it is vital that reactions to rape are understood so that they can be taken into account appropriately. Victims can then be reassured that their reactions are perfectly normal.

A second important advance has been the publication of the Conservative government's 'Victim's Charter' in 1990 which set out principles of good practice so as to put the care and welfare of victims of crime at the centre of the investigative process. A campaign to get these implemented successfully was launched in 1995 with the publication of the rights of victims of crime police paper (Victim Support 1995). These rights were grouped under five main headings: to be free of the burden of decisions relating to the offender; to receive information and explanation about the progress of the case and to have the opportunity to provide their own information about the case for use in the criminal justice process; to be protected in any way necessary; and to receive compensation and to receive respect, recognition and support. In 1991 the Home Office published the Victim's Charter in which criminal justice agencies were asked to re-assess services to victims.

We are only now beginning to understand more about the experiences of women who report rape or indecent assault to the police. Three studies, however, have thrown some light on recent improvements in police practice and their limitations. In Temkin's (1996) very thorough study of the experiences of twenty-three women who reported rape to the Sussex police between 1991 and 1993, she focused on three aspects: their reactions to police processes at every stage from reporting to the trial; their overall attitudes; and finally those aspects of their experience which were particularly positive or negative. The results were compared with the questionnaire study undertaken by Adler (1991). Secondly, Victim Support (1996) carried out a survey of 92 Victim Support schemes and 17 witness services which had supported 938 and 590 victims respectively during 1995. An evaluation study was also conducted by the Northumbria reach project (Maddock and Scott 1996) when eleven women who had reported rape to the police were interviewed. The Northumbria REACH developed from an alliance with the Tyneside Rape Crisis Centre and the Northumbria police.

## The Islington study

Forty women responded to the letter, some 12 per cent of those to whom the letter was sent. It is likely that there were important reasons why some women were not prepared to be interviewed. Ten of these women wrote to tell us that they would find it too painful. Most of them had gone to court and the suspect had been found not guilty. The reasons they gave for not speaking to us are a moving testimony to the pain they had experienced and wanted so desperately to forget. It is significant that none of the defendants in these cases had been convicted and several cases had been 'no crimed'. The following are typical of the replies:

> I just to try and forget what happened. (From a woman who had gone to court and the defendant, an acquaintance, had been found not guilty of rape and ABH.)

> I am just getting over the assault and do not wish to discuss the matter, because it is still painful to do so. (From another woman allegedly raped by her ex-boyfriend who was found not guilty at the Crown Court.)

> I am finding it hard to cope and do not want to go through any questions that will remind me of what happened. I'm sorry. (From a case of alleged attempted rape that had been 'no crimed' on the grounds that the woman was a prostitute. The police report reads 'Prostitute agreed to have sex for £20, apparently changed her mind'.)

> Because I would like to put the past behind me. (From a woman whose case of attempted rape was 'no crimed'.)

> Thank you for your concern but I would like it if it was not brought up again. Many thanks again. (Case of woman who was indecently assaulted which was not taken to court because of 'insufficient evidence'.)

> I do not want to take part. Bringing back memories, suffering shock, paranoia, nightmares although it might help me to get support. I'm surviving. (From a woman whose case went to court but the defendant was also found not guilty.)

> Do not want to take part because it is forgotten about. (Case 'no crimed'.)

Twenty-eight women wrote to say they were willing to be interviewed. Two of those contacted cancelled the appointment on three occasions and failed to answer a letter inviting them for another interview. Therefore twenty-six women were interviewed, two on the telephone, as they indicated that they would find a face to face interview too distressing. Nine of these said they had been victims of rape or attempted rape. In addition, two local women who had reported rape were contacted through a newspaper article that we placed in the local paper. These two had been raped by strangers. All the interviews were recorded, transcribed and analyzed.

Nine women from the Islington police survey, who said they had been victims of rape or attempted rape, were interviewed. In three cases the offence had been initially recorded as rape or attempted rape, but later reclassified (in two cases as indecent assault and in the other case it had been 'no crimed'). In Lizzie's case the suspect, described as tall and blond, was already on an eighteen month suspended sentence. He had waited in the lobby of her block of flats and had jumped on her naked when she returned from an evening out, thrown her to the ground, and with his penis erect, tried to rape her. She had managed to get away, but, in spite of the circumstances, the case was classified as indecent assault. In the second case Una had been raped by her husband from whom she was separated and who was already subject to an injunction. The charge had been reduced to indecent assault and ABH. The indecent assault charge had not been upheld in court and he was only found guilty of ABH. The case of a young black woman whom we have called Cree involved an ex-boyfriend, who had allegedly held her prisoner for several hours and raped her; the case had been 'no crimed'.

*Table 6.1* Details of eleven women interviewed who reported rape or attempted rape

| | |
|---|---|
| 1 rape (Jenny) by stranger (housebreaking) | Guilty: 8 years |
| 1 attempted rape (Amanda) by stranger (taken into consideration with a further rape) | Guilty: 6 years |
| 1 attempted rape (Nora) by stranger (housebreaking) | Guilty: 8 years |
| 2 rapes (Fiona and Anna) by strangers | Suspect not identified |
| 2 attempted rapes (Sharon, Jacky aged 72) by strangers | Suspect not identified |
| 1 attempted rape (Lizzie) by stranger (reclassified as IA, 2 other offences TIC) | Guilty of IA: 3 years |
| 1 attempted rape (Carolyn by acquaintance and theft of £100) | Acquitted |
| 1 rape of intimate (Una) reclassified as IA and ABH | Guilty of ABH |
| 1 rape (Cree) by intimate | 'No crimed' |

Regarding the relationship between the assailant and the victim, seven had been attacked by strangers; two, Cree and Una, by an intimate (men with whom they had had a sexual relationship); and two by an acquaintance. Four of those (Amanda, Nora, Sharon and Jacky) attacked by strangers had fought their assailants off. These are the cases most likely to be reported to the police. Another feature of three of the four cases is that violence was either used or threatened. In two cases the men had actually used a knife in each attack, and in the third case the man had tried to strangle the victim. Without this violence these cases might well have not been reported. In another case (Fiona) involving an actual rape, the suspect was never identified. In one of the two cases contacted through the newspaper, in which Jenny's house was broken into, the defendant was convicted and in the other case (Anna), the defendant was never found.

There are two significant factors about this sample of cases of rape and attempted rape. Most important is that only three of the complainants had been assaulted by someone known to them. In all three cases the police had clearly not taken them as seriously as the others. One case had been 'no crimed' and, in the case of marital rape the charge had been reduced to indecent assault. Carolyn's case had only reached court because the defendant had stolen a hundred pounds from her. Carolyn had met the suspect on the night in question and gone back to his lodging for a coffee. He had attacked her and she had fled leaving the money she had just received from her father behind. This was the main reason she reported the attack although she had suffered injuries. The defendant was acquitted.

Other significant features of the sample are that four of them had fought their attackers off and only a small proportion of women who had been raped were prepared to be interviewed. In one of the three attempted rape cases the suspect had been arrested for other sexual offences. Amanda, whose case had been recorded as attempted rape, had been severely beaten up on her way to work at 9 a.m. A widow, living on her own with two children aged 8 and 10, she was attacked eighteen months after her husband had died. She appeared a very well balanced mature woman and had fought her attacker off vigorously, screaming at the top of her voice: 'You are not going to rape the mother of my children'. In this case the suspect had been charged with a subsequent rape against another woman some months later, and the attempted rape of Amanda had been taken into consideration, so she had not had to appear as a witness. In the second case, the defendant had been caught red handed. Nora awoke to find a man on her bed who had broken into the house, threatened her with a knife and tried to rape her. He had been overpowered by her husband who responded to her screams. Finally, in the case of Jacky, aged 72, the assailant was never apprehended.

The women varied in age from 17 to 72 years old, and came from varied social class and ethnic backgrounds. Occupations were varied; the women included a secretary, a van driver, a social worker, a translator, a fund-raiser for a charity, a teacher, a student, office workers, hostel wardens and hotel workers, a highly successful manager and a voluntary work manager. All but one was working. Over half were married, mostly with children, one was a single parent, and the others were young single women mainly living on their own. Two of the women had only reported cases of indecent assault because the police actually observed the offences taking place. Despite the small size of the sample, it did include women from different racial and ethnic groups. Two of those interviewed were Afro-Caribbean, one was Asian and the rest were white, two from Ireland and one from France.

A further three women had gone to the police when they had been assaulted a second time after a rape that they had not initially reported. Jane, for example, had been raped by her ex-husband and had not reported it. Some years later she had then been assaulted on the street by a stranger and this time had gone to the police. Carol, aged 21, had been raped by her boyfriend with whom she had not wanted to have a sexual relationship. She was a virgin and had told no-one, breaking off her relationship immediately with the young man concerned. The experience had had a devastating effect on her life and she had since stopped going out at night. Returning from work some months later, she had been followed home and grabbed in the street by a man who had indecently assaulted her. She had been terrified and this time had reported the case to the police.

### Effects of assaults on all 26 victims

The complainants who had been raped or subjected to violent attacks all experienced effects which reflected similar findings to the research conducted on what has been described as the 'rape trauma syndrome'. Some women who had suffered less serious attacks also suffered from sleeplessness, nightmares, fear of going out alone and fear of being alone. Two women who had been the victims of minor attacks, involving in one case her breast being grabbed, and in another her bottom being touched, had both reported the cases because the police had actually observed what had happened and urged the women that they should take the case to court. It is probable that neither of them would have bothered to report the cases if the police had not been there to arrest the man. These two cases provided a base line from which to judge reactions.

Brenda was a very successful woman, who was used to taking a great deal of responsibility chairing meetings and holding a responsible post in local government. Three years before the interview, she had suffered an attack one afternoon while out shopping with her daughter. A man had grabbed both her breasts as she had crossed the road at the traffic lights and then run off. By chance two police officers in a car, which had stopped at the lights, had observed what had happened and the man had been arrested. Brenda describes her reaction:

> It shook me up a lot, more than I think I realize. It's strange when I cross roads even now. I'm always checking to see there is not someone coming towards me and I do it on the street and for a long time I did not actually cross the road. I mean I think I'm quite organized and strong and yet I noticed that for a long time I walked down the street much more aware of my surroundings than before. It just makes you very wary. Most people think there's a bit of space around us which people only come past if you invite them and by somebody just forcing themselves on you. I mean it's like you have to watch that nobody else is going to do it.

She was surprised by the effect of the assault. Three years later she could remember little of her activities at the time, but had a clear memory of the man's hands:

> I can't think of anything else that I could tell you and describe at all. I think you do one of two things with difficult incidents. You either block them out completely or else they remain crystal clear. I don't think there is any point in describing it to a man because I don't think they would understand any of it. They don't have breasts and therefore they don't understand the significance of them. They are part of your whole sexual self. I suppose I always thought beforehand that you could pick yourself up and say right, you know, let's carry on.

Jane, who suffered a minor attack, thinks it would have been worse if she had been attacked by someone she knew. She did not therefore think she could be blamed:

I was just lucky I didn't have the typical victim's aftermath, feeling guilty, really dirty and with all my clothes and everything. Well I think that stemmed from the fact that I didn't know the guy. Had it been local or a past boyfriend or something like that, then I think it would have been a lot different. I could genuinely see I didn't give him the come on or anything.

Jenny, victim of an appalling attack by a man who had broken into her house and raped her relentlessly for three hours, said she had never returned to the flat and had been homeless for three years afterwards. She described the effect:

It changes your life for ever, from feeling free and liberal, to feeling trapped. It's like a total loss of independence. I used to walk the streets at 5 a.m. Now I'm too scared to go out at all. After the trial everyone thinks it's all over, but that is when the real panic sets in. It is something you think about every day of your life. It is endless. It has taken me years to recover enough to work again. I went home for three months, although I'd left six years before.

Amanda, also attacked by a stranger, in spite of fighting off her assailant, still blamed herself and was unable to go out for a long while after the attack. She said that because it happened at nine o'clock in the morning, she did not ever feel safe and took taxis everywhere. She also described the common tendency to self-blame:

I'm very very nervous when I'm out and you get this idea like 'I am a victim', like having a sign on my back saying 'attack me'. This feeling I held for weeks; I remember having this awful feeling that 'It's my fault'. It's a very strange feeling. You can't intellectualize it. It's an emotional thing. It's there, it really is. 'I am one of life's victims, treat me as such.'

My reaction was very strange, because it was between total rage, anger, fury and hate to the opposite, of feeling nothing. Because he wasn't brutal like the coarse horrible man you'd expect a rapist to be. Also because he talked calmly and he bargained: He said 'If you don't scream I won't stick the knife into you.' When you imagine rape, you don't expect even to hear his voice.

Like Amanda, most women were taken aback by the effect attacks had on them. For example Sharon, who was attacked in the hallway of her block of flats one afternoon when she was returning home with her 9-year-old son Jim, said:

> I think I trivialized it in my mind. In the back of my mind was this idea that I had to keep everything together for Jim. He didn't understand what the attack was about, and kept saying he did not know why the man had not taken my bag. Really I should have flipped my lid and had a couple of gins and stayed in bed with some tranquillisers and not gone to work. Instead I behaved very oddly. It really coloured my life.

Her reaction was delayed as is so often the case with women suffering from rape trauma syndrome. She reacted by becoming very depressed some months later:

> I had always been a sociable person and all of a sudden I had no motivation whatsoever and I felt that everything was a real effort and I just couldn't go out with my friends. I drank a lot also. I used to like a social glass of wine but I really did start to drink heavily especially during the Christmas period. I am wary about going out. When I come in the flat entrance I wonder whether to take the lift or run up the stairs. I try not to think about someone breaking in the house. You should feel safe in your own four walls.

The whole family is often affected by sexual assault. Sharon described the effect on her relationship with her son:

> It certainly has affected our relationship. He used to see me as this big strong person who made things happen and then he saw me floored literally. But he also kept saying that he couldn't do anything and he still feels that he didn't protect me. And he saw me vulnerable as well. Then there was the time we had an argument about something I wouldn't let him do, and he shoved me and I went right across the kitchen. I don't know whether he was copying the man but he must have realized that I could be physically overpowered where normally children think that the parent can't be overpowered regardless of how big or small they are. I went absolutely mad.

In the case of marital rape, the effect on children is known to be very damaging. Una, who had been raped by her husband, also described the effect on the children:

I even took them to Child Guidance. They really went through it and had trouble at school and everything. That was really upsetting and you often think you shouldn't put kids through it but you have to get rid of the problem. It's worth the aggravation and trauma in the end.

Typical reactions included taking time off work, fear of travelling, low self-esteem, and breaking up sexual relationships. Extra expense was often involved. Six women gave up courses or left their work. Dina, an Asian woman, who was the victim of what is described as 'breast grabbing' was traumatized by it:

I was not recovering for a very long time. I never took my clothes off even when I was married and the kind of intimacy of someone touching me made me very angry. It happened before where someone passed by and touched my bottom and I've always felt angry about things like that, but I distance them. But with this I couldn't get rid of the feeling of the hand. For a long time afterwards I couldn't go that way and I had to give up my course in teacher training. I went back a year later. I still get the feeling but not as badly as before.

Madeleine had been working as a caretaker when one of the men renting rooms had sexually assaulted her. She had also given up being in charge of the house afterwards. All the women interviewed felt less safe when travelling. One woman bought a bicycle and another only took minicabs when she knew the driver. One complainant explained how she felt: 'It comes back. I notice that whenever I was coming back from the tube I would be looking around all the time. I would have to walk on the other side of the road to any man'.

The feeling that they were overreacting was a common response:

I felt I was over reacting. I could have been dead or it could have lasted longer than it did. I know women who have had much worse experiences with pain and things like that. I think 'Do I have the right to feel this bad about it?' And you don't know because different things affect different people in different ways and at different times. It is such a hidden subject. You just don't know whether you are justified in feeling as you do. You don't know whether you are being weak. It's a bit like bereavement because you've lost part of yourself.

Some women had more severe reactions and had taken time off work, and were scared of ever going out. The following young woman, Tina, only 19 years old, had been assaulted minutes after her boyfriend had caught a bus within a short distance of her home:

I had time off then, a week that's what happened. I was on anti-depression tablets even now the effects of it, you know I don't, can't really go out. It changed me completely, I was sick for a long time after that. I thought I'd lose my job. I was off work all the time. I mean once something like that happens to you, it just gets you down. You're run down and you're just open for everything. I had the flu all the time. I wasn't sleeping. I was always having nightmares. I still have nightmares till this day, every now and again, not as often as I did, but I have nightmares about it. I wake in a sweat. I think it was quite bad that I wasn't offered any support really, and as far as I'm concerned they knew that I didn't have any sort of record.

Few people have any idea of how traumatic rape can be and how long term are the effects, although reactions vary as the following account reveals:

I don't think I'd be able to handle it if it happened to me again. I mean it's not as bad as other people but it was bad enough. Not being able to sleep, taking depression tablets, the shakes. I had to go to the doctor. They told me to go, to get it put down on my record. So I went to the doctor and they put me on tablets.

A number of complainants left their jobs and moved house. This 26-year-old woman who had left her job and moved house, bravely devised a programme of recovery for herself:

But then it was afterwards a couple of weeks later it kind of got to me. It was coming back to me that I didn't have anywhere to live, I didn't have a job to go to. I worked out a programme of recovery for myself and the first thing I did was, I went back to where it happened during the day and the second thing was walking out at night with a friend, because walking out at night absolutely terrified me. Then the third stage was walking out alone by myself and I'd given up completely on fellas at that stage and I said 'Right, just get on with work and everything and take things gradually and don't rush into a relationship, nothing like that'.

Four complainants feared further attack or retaliation from men who were charged with offences. Tina described how her cousin who had witnessed the attack had been threatened.

> My cousin, they were threatening her over ten months. She wouldn't give evidence. She ended up going back to Ireland. So it would have been my word against his at the end of the day. On one against one I wouldn't have stood a chance. I was very angry with her. I'll never speak to her again.

Nora, who had screamed so loudly that her husband had come and fought off the attacker, had suffered from long-term effects. Three years after the attack she said:

> My sleep pattern is so bad that I can't stay anywhere else, can I? I mean I get up and walk around all night, put the television on all night and you can't do that in other people's houses. It's not fair.

Complainants described the way that being raped had had a long-term influence on their lives. Anna said:

> I've become far more mistrusting. Much more sceptical about the motivation in my relationships with other men. I've become much more cautious about the things I do and the way I dress. I never wear skirts now because I just don't feel comfortable in them. I think I've become a lot more aggressive as well.

Sexual problems are common and it is not unusual for relationships to break up as Linda explained:

> It must have been a year after that I went out with someone else and that was really hard. It was awful. I just didn't trust him at all. In fact looking back on it the only reason that I really went out with him was to prove to myself that I wasn't terrified of men and it was a disaster. I think I had to go through with it being the first person since it had happened. He didn't understand at all. He was always pressuring me into sex and that just made it worse.

Partners were not always understanding of such reactions. Rodkin *et al.* (1982) observed partners' reactions when running a support group for male relatives of rape victims. Men initially responded like the victims themselves, showing fear reactions and then often became very protective and spent more time with their partner. They often blamed themselves for not providing adequate protections. At a later stage, they became irritated with the length of time it took women to recover and resented their partner's dependency. Often women could not bear to be touched. This led men to withdraw into work, which was often interpreted by the women as rejection. Relatives often felt overwhelmed with helplessness and needed help in coming to terms with the assault.

Several researchers have found a close connection between recovery and short- and long-term support (Holmstrom and Burgess 1978). Maguire and Corbett (1987) found that friends and volunteers such as Victim Support and Rape Crisis were only partly helpful and intimates were far the most crucial in determining long-term recovery.

### *Attitudes to police treatment*

A distinction should be made in comparing the satisfaction of complainants with their treatment by female and male police officers during the investigatory side of the procedure and the taking of a statement. Roughly three-quarters (20 out of 28) of the women interviewed were broadly satisfied with the way they were treated by the women police officers. They appreciated the increase in the number of female officers dealing with cases of sexual assault, and some were surprised that the police treated their complaint so seriously and sympathetically.

> I don't usually trust the police at all but they were great. It seemed as though it was really important to them. They really did make me feel supported the whole way through.

> I never had the slightest undercurrent that anybody didn't believe me. I felt one hundred per cent supported by everybody. It didn't seem like anyone was acting and believing anything different to what I had told them.

> The police woman was very gentle in her approach and we just talked about it before she took the statement and she let me know what was coming. She was very gentle in that way. I didn't feel interrogated at all.

> They couldn't have been nicer and my friend came and both she and the WPC didn't smoke but I was smoking like a chimney

because I was a nervous wreck. The poor souls. They were so kind.

The nicest point was at the end when the WPC actually said 'Thank you for coming and reporting it'. She was telling me about the number of situations that are not reported and that women don't actually think they are severe enough to report. But it's people like that who may turn out to be rapists. Just to think that his name is on the computer now so when anything happens, they'll knock on his door. She said that if he's been warned like that then the chances are it will put him off from doing it again because he can't get away with it anymore.

Some male detectives were also praised. Fiona, raped by a stranger, had nothing but praise for the detective who handled her case:

He was really lovely. He was in his forties, real family man and everything. He came across like he was really caring and really sympathetic. He just wanted to make sure that basically I was OK. He said the office was open any time I wanted to have a word with him and he really meant it. He just seemed to be this really lovely father figure more than anything else. We got on really well.

Jacky, aged 72, fully appreciated the officers whom she said had come round the moment she rang and kept in touch with her: 'They are my best friends' she commented. After the attempted rape, they often rang to find out how she was. 'No-one will ever run a copper down to me' she said. She was asked to come down to the station to an identification parade but she refused as she said she was too afraid of picking out the wrong person. In terms of improvements she did not think the police could have behaved better.

Four out of the eleven complainants who had been victims of rape or attempted rape were dissatisfied with the male police officers who had dealt with their cases. Their dissatisfaction concerned either the effectiveness of the police response, which was sometimes inappropriate, delayed or inefficient, or the way they were treated by the police. The most serious complaints involved victims feeling that they were not believed and had been treated with suspicion.

Nora, aged 52, was appalled by the fact that the police had disbelieved her. She gave an account of the classic stranger rape nightmare, in which the police appear to have disbelieved her, actually accusing her sick husband of attacking the intruder.

I woke up and this man was all over me and he had a knife at my neck and I can't go into much detail because it still really bothers me and I still get nightmares about it. I think it's getting worse to be honest. First I thought it was a nightmare and I thought 'I wish I'd hurry up and wake up'. Then I realized it wasn't a nightmare and it was really happening. The terror, no-one can describe it, it was so awful and then I screamed and he said 'Don't make a sound or you're dead'. It was just natural for me to scream and I never thought about the consequences at the time. I couldn't move I don't know why. I just screamed and screamed and then my husband came in and he put the light on and he was just so shocked. He was ill as well. Then I saw the knife and it was a great big meat knife. My face was cut and I've still got scars.

Her house was broken into in the middle of the night. She was threatened with rape at knife point and only saved by her husband's bravery. The man had cut her husband's arms, but had been disarmed by him. Her husband was ill with lung cancer and was sleeping in a different room. (He has since died.) She described what happened when the police arrived:

The police went downstairs and I don't know how much time elapsed but they came up and said 'Do you realize how serious a charge this is? He (the defendant) said he had met you in a pub and that your husband had come in and found you in bed together'. I couldn't believe they really seemed to believe him. I was so disgusted and my husband said 'I beg your pardon'. They said 'You should only use reasonable force'. My husband said 'What you're telling me is that he broke into my home, attacked my wife and you're telling me that we shouldn't use force'. But they said it was a serious charge and I said 'I don't know what you think because I don't go to pubs'. I suppose if it had been some sort of woman who went to pubs, he would have got off with it.

She tried to understand why they had reacted in this way:

I've got nothing against the police but it's what they stand for. They're not really fair, are they? I realize they get people who lie, but you don't expect the police to believe that I met him in a pub and we were caught in bed together. I mean me a 50-year-old woman with a boy of 26. I mean my son's older than him and the state of him. He stunk. I'll never get over it. It was absolutely

awful. I thought he'd have to kill me. I didn't think of the consequences.

Nora had only agreed to be interviewed in the hope that it would
lead to an improvement in police practice.

> I mean I'll never forget that never. For somebody to break into
> your home and attack you and then, you call the police and they
> tell you that you're lying and that they had to warn me that it was
> a very serious offence to lie. This was after I had been abused and
> touched and grovelled all over. My husband came out with a load
> of swear words that I had never heard him use. Well, the mind
> boggles to think about it. That did stick in my mind. I don't think
> the police have got much regard for people. I really don't think
> they were very helpful. I think their attitude needs changing.

Amanda, a widow with two children who had been the victim of a
nasty stranger attack occurring in broad daylight, was taken to a
police station and felt like a criminal:

> When you're brought into the police station past the desk where
> all the criminals come in and all the police are wandering around.
> I felt like a criminal not a victim. You know you have that little
> guilt bit thinking 'I am a victim' you know but I just didn't feel
> comfortable being taken in by a load of policemen to the station.
> So they need more discretion.

She also resented the fact that the police had checked up on her. This
unnerved her. She describes how she felt:

> This policeman knew about me and it really took me aback that
> they had checked up on me. I suppose they had looked in some
> police files. Excuse my paranoia. They must have done because
> they knew I was from Glasgow. It was a surprise to me as if they
> were somehow questioning my word.

She was, however, full of praise for the woman police officer who had
taken her statement. When asked what she was like she replied:
'Absolutely marvellous. I can't speak highly enough of her. She even
gave me her phone number and said I could contact her anytime'.
However, she was never informed about what happened to her case
although her attacker had been arrested and convicted of another

rape. She had tried to find out but to no avail, and the original police woman had moved.

In a case involving a young black woman, Cree, whose allegation of rape was 'no crimed', she explained how she had lost confidence in the police after the accused was freed the same day and the case dropped. She had not even been informed. It is perhaps significant that both Cree and her alleged assailant were known to each other and were black.

Una, the victim of domestic violence, had mixed feelings about the police. She had had great difficulty in getting the police to come to the house although she felt her life had been in danger; she had rung the police previously on a number of occasions when she said all they had done was 'give him [her estranged husband] a little talking to and leave'. She was disappointed in how long it had taken to arrest her husband:

> I have to say it took two calls to get them there and when they got there and saw how bad I looked they were really sorry that they didn't realize how serious it was. I was quite knocked up with a lot of bruises and cuts. The other thing that disappointed me was how long it took to arrest him. It felt as though it wasn't important enough. If he had assaulted someone else they would have arrested him straight away and that really annoyed me He was all cocky and said he wasn't worried about the injunction. He got a bit of a shock when he realized I meant what I said.

On the other hand, she had been impressed with they way 'the coppers are changing their attitudes more now' and had decided to join the police herself: 'The whole experience made me want to join the police. I thought that is what I want to do'.

Seven women had mixed views of the police. They were upset by some of the questions the police asked. Three women objected to questions about what they were wearing. Bridget who had been attacked in broad daylight when returning home with her young son from school said:

> One of the things I did think was awful was when I had to make a statement and the WPC said herself that she hated having to ask me but 'What was I wearing?' I just thought 'What the bloody hell difference does it make?'

Such questions are, of course, asked in court as Sylvia described: 'The magistrate wanted to know what I was wearing. I told them trainers, jeans and a jacket. Hardly the sort of thing that was outrageous'. The police presumably see such questions as preparation for court. Additionally, police sometimes asked questions about the past sexual history and life style of complainants which were not relevant and then could be used by defence lawyers against them.

Eight women in our research were critical of the police methods of investigation. Two of these had reported indecent assault, but where the suspect had not been identified. They were unimpressed with the police and had had difficulty in even finding out how to report the crimes. One of these women had had to go to two police stations. She contrasted this with when she had reported a burglary and the police had come round immediately:

> Strange that I could not report it at the police station nearest my house. They said it was because it was another area's offence. I might well not have bothered. If I hadn't had a bike I wouldn't have reported it.

Two other women were critical of the offhand way the police had reacted to their report. They did not think that a serious attempt had been made to arrest the suspect. Natasha, a confident married woman in her early thirties, had been assaulted on her way home from the tube station one rainy night and had called the police immediately. They had not pursued the suspect although Natasha had given them a very clear description. The only further contact she had had was ten days later:

> They (the police) called me and they said: 'The young man that assaulted you. We think we know who he is. He lives locally, he's done it before. We've had it reported eight times in the past year, providing we are talking about the same bloke. In every case the attack was very similar. The physical description is very similar, so we think we are talking about the same bloke. He's never actually raped, and we don't have a good enough description to pin him down.' They said the file was still open.

She was surprised that as there had been so many attacks, the police had not thought it worth while to bring her in to go through some photokits. She did not think the offences were being taken seriously enough.

In the second case the suspect had actually been arrested, but there had not been any follow up. Dina describes what happened:

I was walking along the road one morning at about 8.30 am and this black bloke blocked my path and grabbed me. My immediate reaction was to swing my arm round to hit him and I shouted abuse at him. I don't know what he did because I was off. I ran to the end of the alley and straight to the police station which was nearby. The police got a panda car and drove to the other end of the alley. He was still there shouting obscenities and they picked him up. They took him back to the station. He fitted my description and I made a statement....They said they wanted me to do an identity parade so that I could pick him out. I suggested they did it soon while I still remembered what he looked like. It really annoyed me that they never came back to me about it. I don't know if he was charged or whatever.

### Attitudes to race

In five of the eleven cases of rape or attempted rape where the victims were interviewed, the suspect was black, in one case both the complainant and suspect were black and in the others both were white. There was therefore a considerable over-representation of black suspects.

Race was an issue that several of the complainants brought up even when their assailant had been white. Two women were offended that the police and other people assumed that the suspect was black:

The police were saying 'Was he black or white?' And I told them he was white and one of them turned round and said 'Makes you ashamed to be white, doesn't it?' They were so upset about it.

So many people said to me 'Was he black?' And in the end I felt embarrassed to say 'Yes' because it would open up everybody's racism. I started to get scared of seeing young black men on the street which is something I was never afraid of. I was used to spending time with the black community around. It really turned on racism in me which I didn't like.

A number of white women were concerned about the racial over-tones of the attack and were concerned that the police would overreact. Anna commented: 'It could so easily be seen as my being anti-black. This was one reason why I found it very difficult to think about going to the police'. She also recognized that there might well have been racial aspects to the attack:

I don't know how to say this without sounding racist myself. But I think it was partly a status thing, to have done that to a white woman was so much more a show of strength than to have done it to a black woman. Because it destroyed my dignity and in a perverse way there must have been an element of racism on their part.

One complainant was glad that her assailant was white because she did not want to contribute to the prejudice that all rapists were black. She said 'I think I would still have reported it if he was black but I would have been sorry to add to that prejudice.'

Another complainant described how she had developed a fear of all men, but particularly of black men, showing the deep rootedness of the stereotype of the black rapist.

It's really weird because the guy was white and English and before I would talk to anybody, it didn't matter who he was as long as he was nice I'd talk to him. But afterwards I couldn't be in a room with a fella alone, there was no way. The first time I went down to Kenny's room we were just talking, but going down there I was shaking. He was sensitive enough to know that something had happened and he guessed what had happened. The only fellas I would see would be gay men. If I was walking down the street and a black guy was coming up towards me, even now I'd be shaking. I honestly don't know why. It's as if this switch has suddenly clicked in my mind and if there's a bunch of white guys coming towards me I'm fine, but if a bunch of black fellas I just seize up completely.

Audrey, who had fought off her assailant, whom she described as black and 'a nice looking fellow, very trendily dressed', thought that her boyfriend would have found it much harder to handle the rape of his girlfriend by a black than a white man. She had not realized before how racist people still are:

I reflected a lot on white men's attitudes to black men and white women with black men. I think if I had been raped by him other (white) men would have been unsympathetic. Sympathetic to my being hurt but I can imagine that it would have made them feel quite outraged and the reaction men feel toward black men is quite strong. It would be utter revulsion from the boyfriend who'd be disgusted by what had happened – ultra disgusting if his girlfriend had been raped by a black man. That would be harder to handle. It would be as hard as if he were the victim.

Two complainants described how the defendants had used racism as an argument against them. On the other hand some defendants played on the myth in their defence that white women find black men sexually irresistible. Jenny, raped by a black man who had broken into her house and raped her for three hours, described a horrific court ordeal. The first trial had resulted in a hung jury and in the second trial the defendant had sacked his counsel and taken on his own defence. The judge had actually made a speech to say that the jury 'should have sympathy for the defendant who has had no legal experience'. Jenny commented:

> The racial aspect was strong. He (the assailant) shouted 'You like black men, you hate black men, your boyfriend is black'. Why should I have to be told that I am a whore and all sorts of inarticulate rubbish in front of all sorts of people? I was furious that this guy is screaming all this abuse.

### Police follow-up

Several women commented on the poor flow of information on the progress of their case; many received no information whatsoever. There appears to be a serious communication gap occurring across the spectrum of case outcomes, although we have no way of knowing whether there was a similar pattern of experiences among the women who declined to be interviewed. It is possible that the most dissatisfied group were the least willing to come forward, especially as our letter was sent to them by the police. In only two of the cases in our study which had gone to court, were complainants satisfied with the contact the police had maintained with them.

In some cases complainants were more satisfied. For example, Fiona, whose case did not, however, reach court, described the police in very positive terms:

> They were always there. They kept me informed. They were always into making sure the victim was informed and not forgotten about and left to feel that nothing was being done. That was really good.

They never caught the guy, but that wasn't their fault. They did what they could. They hunted for three years.

Fiona thought she may have been kept in touch because she was the 'genuine article', i.e. a respectable girl, with a job and a boyfriend, who had been raped by a stranger and had developed a good relationship with the detective inspector.

Far more common, however, in cases involving acquaintances or less serious assaults than actual rape, complainants were not always even told the outcome of the investigation. This caused anxiety and made women feel it was not worth reporting:

After I reported it I didn't really hear anything about it and I thought 'What's going on here?' You know I've never been to court, I didn't know what would happen.

I couldn't go through all that being put through to so many people before you get the information you wanted. (From a woman who had been the victim of attempted rape and GBH.)

I never heard anything about it again. (From a woman who experienced an attack where she fought off the young man.)

The only important thing to me is that I didn't know what had happened afterwards. That would be my main complaint, that someone should have given me a ring. (See Dina above.)

Apart from the assault in my very own street, I have also been mugged three times. In all cases nothing has come of it. I was never informed of results plus or minus, waste of time. (This was in a case where in fact the suspect was taken to court and received one month's imprisonment.)

The police telephoned me on one occasion a couple of months later. They had somebody for doing something similar and asked if I could come in if they needed me. I said I would come immediately but they never did call me again.

Even 'genuine articles' were not necessarily kept in touch. In Amanda's case, a health service professional, who as we have seen experienced an attempted rape, was not informed of the outcome of her case even after it had gone to court. The defendant had actually raped another woman and her case had been taken into consideration so she did not need to go to court. The police wrote to her telling her the case would be going to court, but never informed her of the outcome. She described her reaction:

> They wrote to me and told me the man had been charged and that I shouldn't leave London without informing the police. That was the first time I saw his name and I started going through the telephone directory. Fortunately I was unable to find him. I did ring quite a few people but I didn't pursue it. I would have hung up if it had been him. I pulled myself together after five or six calls. I said to myself 'This is the reaction of the paranoiac, now put it behind you'. I never heard what happened. I'd like to have known if he got jailed or fined. I'd like to know if he usually did this sort of thing or whether it was a one off. They did say they would let me know which gives me the feeling that nothing has actually happened.

In this case we were able to tell her that the suspect had received a seven-year prison sentence. This indicates that even in the few cases that reach court the complainant is not necessarily told what happens. It seems quite extraordinary that the police do not realize the effect this has and discomfort it causes. This is an area which needs urgent attention.

Another area of concern is that even if more women find out when the assailant has been sentenced, they are rarely told when they are going to be released. As Amanda explained:

> Sometimes women are told that the man's gone to prison but then they're not told about when they are going to be released. It's a whole area that people don't think about, especially after the case. Again it is a question of money and caring for the victim. There should be some sort of agency responsible for this, preferably not the police. Just for making sure there is after care and support for the victim.

Nora, whose case is mentioned above, was upset that her bedding was never returned: 'They took away all my bedding, my nightwear, my housecoat, everything I had on. Not that you want it back. But I never got an offer. It was a brand new quilt and pillow cases'. This illustrates the total invasion of privacy that reporting a rape involves, where even her bedding and clothing are whipped away for testing.

In Adler's (1991) study this was the area of police practice that came under the most criticism. Her respondents did not think that they were told enough about the whole process of investigation, and were not given enough information about why they had to undergo the various medical and investigatory procedures. Nor were they always told about the outcome of cases. For example, some women were not told when the suspect was arrested, what crime he was charged with, let alone when he was to be released. In our study likewise, we have seen how little information complainants were given. None of the complainants was told when a suspect was going to be released after serving a prison sentence. This was an area of particular concern where women feared that the assailant would return to punish them for giving evidence against them, which does happen on occasion. Nora describes this fear:

> What I do worry about is that when he does get out he might come back. I suppose it's stupid really. Your mind does funny things with you at times. I try not to think about it.

Most extreme of all was Sandy's experience. She was not informed that her assailant, who had been sentenced to five years, had been released on appeal. This is the kind of task the police chaperone system will need to take on (discussed below).

## Evidence from recent initiatives

Towards the end of the period of our research, the Metropolitan Police introduced a chaperone system whereby a female officer (or a male officer in the case of assaults on men) who has completed the training programme on Sexual Offences Investigation Techniques, is assigned to a case from the outset and assumes responsibility, as far as possible, for all communication with the complainant. Although a detective inspector (most of whom are male) takes overall charge of the investigation, it is the chaperone who takes the complainant's statement, accompanies her to the medical, assists her in attending a clinic for sexually transmitted diseases and advises her about support services. If it seems unlikely that the case will go to court, the chaperone is required to emphasize that what happened was not the complainant's fault and that it was 'just a problem of evidence'. The chaperone therefore acts as a liaison officer between the investigative team and the victim, and in the longer term she keeps the complainant informed of criminal investigations, prepares her for an identification parade, where necessary, and accompanies her throughout the court proceedings (see Chapter 5 for details of the chaperone's duties). However, the complainants we interviewed had reported before these reforms had been introduced.

The Victim Support interviews (1996), conducted after the chaperone system had been in operation for a number of years, indicate that there is still cause for concern. Ten of the eleven women interviewed in the Victim Support study reported that although the police kept them informed initially, this petered out as the case progressed. They wanted information about trial dates, bail decisions, full details of their injuries, information on medical issues, legal procedures, the outcome of the case, appeal decisions and the offender's release date. Nine of the ten interviewees whose cases went to court mentioned problems in relation to a lack of information on and delays surrounding trial dates. The report recommends that fixed dates and fewer delays are regarded as a priority (ibid. 53). Bail was a particular problem. Victim Support Schemes were asked whether the police usually asked for the victim's views on bail decisions. In February 1995, the Director of Public Prosecutions announced that victims would be consulted on their views but it was not clear whether this was in fact being implemented.

Temkin (1997a), who had undertaken an in-depth study of women's experience of reporting rape in Sussex in 1995, found that force guidelines outlining how officers should deal with rape were only introduced in 1997, and although rape was generally handled by specialist Child Protection Teams, their training concentrated on child abuse and the officers were not available after 10 p.m. At the time there was also only one rape examination suite, although four more have been opened since.

Out of the 57 cases which fitted the study criteria, 30 per cent resulted in interviews, and with the addition of another 6 cases, 23 women were finally interviewed. The relatively small number indicates the difficulty of gaining feedback from rape victims about their experiences. Reasons for refusal were not always stated but included, as in our research, reluctance to have to think about the trauma again. No clear distinction emerged between complainants who agreed to be interviewed and those who refused. Temkin divided her respondents into three groups: those with positive attitudes, those with mixed views and those with negative views. Thirteen of the 23 (57 per cent) were categorized as wholly or mainly positive about their treatment by officers, 7 (30 per cent) as having a mixed response and 3 (13 per cent) were categorized as negative. Therefore two-thirds (20) of the complainants were wholly, mainly or partly positive and a third (10) were wholly, mainly or partly negative about their experiences.

Complainants who were wholly or mainly positive about the police were more likely to have been raped by a stranger (4 out of 13 compared to none in the other categories who had been raped by relatives, friends, acquaintances or employers), more likely to have reported immediately (54 per cent compared to only 2 out of the 10 combined mixed or negative categories) and to have been subjected to violence or threats (in the positive category 69 per cent had sustained external injuries, violence or threats compared to only 20 per cent of the mixed or negative categories). However, most of the women who were wholly or partly positive had been raped by acquaintances, 46 per cent had reported immediately and 31 per cent had not been subjected to violence or threats.

Women who were less satisfied or dissatisfied with police treatment had been raped by acquaintances or intimates. Out of the 10 (5 of whom were under 20) 7 complained that their allegations had been met with disbelief by the police. Temkin reports that the main reason for dissatisfaction was being harshly questioned or treated with disbelief by the police at some stage in the proceedings. What mattered most to victims was to be treated with sympathy, to feel believed and to retain contact with the police and to be kept informed about developments. Temkin concludes that there is still evidence of old-style attitudes towards dealing with women who report rape. She found that as well as women reporting unsympathetic questioning, one woman had received no help when she was harassed by her assailant who had followed her and kept a watch on her home, telephoning her constantly during the night. The police had said that there was not a lot they could do.

Sixteen police officers were also interviewed in her research. Only one had received any training about the effects of rape on victims. Five of the sixteen interviewed (32 per cent) felt that the training they had received was completely inadequate and a further five who had been on the detectives' training course felt that the training neglected victims and concentrated on investigatory techniques. Moreover she found that 'myths' about rape were still widespread. Half of the sixteen officers considered that a quarter of all rapes reported to the police were false. Victims who knew the assailant, reported late and had no injury were still regarded as objects of suspicion. She argues strongly that training should involve challenging the myths of rape and the stereotypes of victims and offenders.

Other research suggests that the police in some areas are improving their response, providing some resources and that at least multi-agency co-ordination has been successfully developed. In Northumbria the

REACH (Rape Examination, Advice, Counselling and Help) project was set up in 1991 to provide a service to women who had been sexually assaulted. It is funded by the Northumbria Police Authority and the local Health Authorities with voluntary input from the Women's Doctors Scheme and support from other agencies. It offers a unique range of services all within the same building. The services provided include: experienced women doctors able to conduct examinations in a purpose-built suite, confidential access to experienced counsellors for a number of sessions regardless of whether or not the woman reports an assault to the police, and specially trained women police officers who can be called on to conduct an interview and take formal statements.

In 1995 the Management Group commissioned an evaluation of the project to gather information about the quality of the service between October 1991 and April 1994 and explore directions for future development and funding. Questionnaires were sent to women complainants and the agencies involved. A total of 149 REACH clients responded to the women's questionnaire, and 36 police officers, 18 doctors and all 5 counsellors responded to the professionals' questionnaires. Sixty-two women who returned the questionnaire were also interviewed, representing 60 per cent of women who had made a statement to the police. The women were asked to rate the police involvement and generally most women rated the service highly. Police and doctors were given a low rating by only two women.

In the evaluation (Maddock and Scott 1995: 27) the main point of criticism from the complainants concerned the lack of communication regarding the progress of their case. The comments indicated that complainants were not always told that defendants were out on bail or had been released and that lack of such information understandably caused great stress.

In our research, in spite of their criticism of the police, the complainants who agreed to be interviewed did not regret reporting it. This is probably not true of some women who had the indignity of seeing the assailant walk free when acquitted. Amanda, who had managed to fight her assailant off, understood how much more difficult it would have been to report actually being raped:

> I think people that I know feel very strongly that you should report to the police. I would never have considered not reporting it. I can understand it if you were raped you wouldn't want to report it though. I think under my circumstances that the children finding out their mother had been raped. My God. I wouldn't want them to have to handle that. They've already had a father die

on them. I wouldn't want them to have a mother who had been raped. So I understand women not going in those circumstances, not through guilt though. I don't think women should not go to the police because of that. You can say 'I'm not guilty.'

According to Detective Inspector Sue Hill of Feltham Police, when interviewed in September 1997, the provision for victims of sexual assault is still *ad hoc*, and it is rather a lottery as to what kind of service victims would receive. She acknowledged that important improvements had been made, but took the view that there were no grounds for complacency. She was somewhat uneasy about the number of male chaperones who were being trained and wondered whether it was really necessary to offer complainants a choice of a female or a male officer to take their statement, when invariably they preferred to talk to a woman. A crucial area was ensuring good communication between the inspector conducting the investigatory side and the chaperone. Lack of communication between them means that the complainant is not always kept in touch with the progress of the case.

Regarding the availability of rape suites, Sue Hill welcomed a move to reduce the absolute number and instead replace them with a few centres of excellence. Many rape suites had not been well maintained and doctors (especially women doctors who were called out at night) were put at some risk in searching for the premises in high crime areas at the dead of night when not familiar with the location. One important innovation was the introduction of quarterly meetings of all officers involved in sexual assault cases to make sure the work load was shared and in order to review their performance. She was concerned that the new personnel policy introduced in 1996 by which uniformed officers are now transferred to the CID and CID officers (after ten years' service) are transferred to the uniformed force, might lead to a less professional service. When, for example, a uniformed officer transferred they were rarely given any training in dealing with sexual offences. She considered there to be a strong argument for a specialist service in this area.

A number of multi-agency projects have been set up to increase inter-agency co-operation around rape and domestic violence. The first of these was the Leeds Inter-agency Project on Women and Violence established in 1989 which was backed by the West Yorkshire Police. Clear guidelines for police officers were developed and a computerized database monitors incidents of violence against women by known men.

## Conclusion

Our research indicates that over the past decade the facilities for dealing with victims have improved. It is no longer necessary, for example, to take the victim through the custody area, but now rape examination suites are available in all areas. Most complainants whom we interviewed were on the whole satisfied with the way they were personally dealt with by the women police. The changes that have been introduced appear to be having a beneficial effect. There was, however, much less satisfaction with the way the case was investigated and followed up. A quarter of the women were still not satisfied with the attitudes of the male police officers investigating their case and pointed to the unsympathetic way they had been treated. The majority were dissatisfied with the lack of follow up by the police. The most widespread dissatisfaction concerned the medical examination, as we shall see in the next chapter.

It should also be borne in mind that only a small proportion of the women who had reported to the police were interviewed and the majority of them had been raped or assaulted by strangers. Such cases are the ones most likely to be taken seriously and treated sympathetically by the police, so that their responses may underestimate the shortcomings of the services. Women who are raped by strangers are also the most likely to report rape to the police, so this type of rape is likely to be over-represented as compared to rapes that occur.

The lack of satisfaction with the investigatory aspects of the service appear to reflect the tendency for assaults not to be taken very seriously. The practice of 'no criming' is still continuing and complainants are also being left with no information as to the outcome of their cases There still appears to be a need for the police to take sexual assaults more seriously and to deal with calls more promptly and effectively.

As Temkin (1997a) argues, there is a vital need for training of the police to take sexual assault more seriously, to deal with it more efficiently and to be aware of the characteristics of rape trauma syndrome so that they have the information they need to enable them to deal more sympathetically with victims of rape. It is significant that police officers described the week's training course at Hendon predominantly in terms of gathering forensic information rather than as developing skills for treating the victims of trauma. Neither Sussex (see Temkin 1997a) nor the Metropolitan CID officers (Adler 1991) had received any training in the understanding of rape trauma syndrome. The Home Office Circular issued to all Chief Constables in response to the call from the Women's National Commission for training of detectives involved with rape, states:

> The attention of chief officers is drawn to the need to ensure that the special needs of victims of rape...are given due weight during appropriate in-force training. In particular, there is a need for investigating officers to understand the different ways in which victims may react and for those officers not to appear to the victims as suspicious or hostile or sceptical.
>
> (Home Office 1986: 3)

Although these guidelines were issued prior to the two year period during which the complainants in our research reported to the police, our findings and Temkin's more recent study highlight the continuing inadequacy of the way victims of sexual assault are treated and demonstrate the urgent need for improvements in police service delivery to women reporting rape and sexual assault.

# 7 Complainants' views: the aftermath of sexual assault

During the 1970s complainants of rape made it clear that the medical examination needed urgent reform (see Smith 1980, Davis 1985, Blair 1985) both in relation to the manner in which it was conducted and the effectiveness with which forensic information was gathered. It appeared that the prejudices of some police surgeons were interfering with the thoroughness of their examinations. For example, Smith (1980: 49) pointed out that surgeons did not always follow up bruising that occurred some time after the attack and many were not aware of the Rape Trauma Syndrome, or the typical symptoms suffered by rape victims. Of the 70 women interviewed by Chambers and Millar (1983), 45 viewed the examination completely negatively and 8 were partly negative. One woman who had been sexually assaulted was even asked if she had enjoyed the experience (ibid. 99–101)! Women complained that the medical procedures were painful and unpleasant and several women described the way they were examined as insensitive, unsympathetic and abrupt (see Temkin 1996).

In regard to where the examination was held, a study by Corbett (1987) in the early 1980s found that most examinations were held in police stations. By 1985 when the Women's National Commission published a report on rape and violence against women, based on a questionnaire study of all police stations, the situation had barely changed. Chief Superintendent Thelma Wagstaff of the Metropolitan Police, in her evidence to the Women's National Commission, explained that examinations were often conducted in a room directly off the charge room where entry and exit could be observed by anyone going in or out (Women's National Commission 1985: paragraph 50).

Following this report and in recognition of the unsuitability of such premises for very vulnerable witnesses, complainants were increasingly examined in doctors' surgeries or special arrangements were made in certain hospitals. Some authorities set up police examinations suites which often served a wide area, and so suffered from the disadvantage that the complainant needed to be transported some distance.

In their 1985 report, the Women's National Commission noted that the Metropolitan Police had agreed to set up eight victim examination suites, and by the end of 1990 this had been accomplished. By 1991, when Adler undertook her survey, only 15 cent of respondents were being examined in police stations. By 1994 three more suites had been added, and victim examination suites had been set up in two hospitals bringing the total number of special facilities in the Metropolitan Police Area to twelve. In Sussex Temkin (1996: 7) interviewed fourteen complainants in 1995, none of whom had been interviewed in a police station. More pessimistically the nationwide Victim Support (1996) report based on interviews with eight complainants who had been medically examined after reporting rape, found that three out of the eight had been examined in a police station. This suggests that country-wide the resources available for sexual assault complainants are still patchy.

Delays in finding a doctor are still a major problem. This was high-lighted in the case of Craig Charles who was acquitted of rape in March 1995. The complainant had to wait 30 hours before she was medically examined as a doctor could not be found. By this time she had washed and there was no DNA evidence available, which appeared to have been a major factor leading to his acquittal (*The Times*, 4 March 1995, Temkin 1996).

## The Islington research

Eleven women interviewed had been medically examined (two of whom had been contacted through the local newspaper). Only two of the eleven were seen by a woman doctor, although all but one had requested to see a woman. The medical examination was described by seven of the women as a stressful experience, some saw it as an endurance test, and three described it as utterly degrading, in one case as bad as the rape itself. Only one woman, who had been exam-ined by a woman doctor, said the examination had been carried out very sympathetically. She described the lady doctor as 'really good' and said that 'she had tried to joke to ease the situation'. Some women had mixed reactions to it. Una, for example, whose allegation of rape was reduced to indecent assault and not held up in court was grateful for the results of the medical although she had found it stressful:

It was OK. In fact it was worth its weight in gold, that medical report. Because he's such a good liar without the report he would have got off on the ABH charge too.

Three doctors appeared to have been callously unsympathetic, even cruel. Others may not have been deliberately heartless, but do not appear to have appreciated the acute sensitivity of victims whose bodies have been abused. Careful thought needs to go into ways of avoiding such degradation. One problem seems to be that the forensic requirements are put into effect with little flexibility. Such descriptions as the following give one little confidence in the service:

So I got examined by the doctor. She wasn't very nice. It was terrible. She gave me the morning after pill and she didn't explain anything about it. I was throwing up – I didn't know I'd be throwing up for nothing. She wasn't the slightest bit sympathetic or anything like that. She didn't care. She was just doing her job.

I looked down at myself with this sheet wrapped around me and he (the medical officer) turned to the WPC and said 'Cover her up will you?' I felt like a piece of something on a slab – cover that up we should not be looking at that.

The presence of the police officer at the examination was seen by some as helpful and by others as distressing. One of the complainants in the REACH study (see previous chapter) found that the presence of a police officer at the medical examination had been very distressing and said she would have preferred the use of a one-way mirror or video (ibid. 31). On the other hand one of the complainants interviewed by Temkin, described the presence of a woman police officer as 'incredible, she was like a best friend'.

In our research, examination by male surgeons came in for stiff criticism. Amanda, herself a medical professional working in a local hospital, was very unhappy with the treatment she had received from the male police surgeon:

The one thing I didn't like was the police surgeon. I don't think the police told him I was the victim and he seemed to treat me as if somehow I was a criminal. I ended up in tears. He just seemed so rude to me, all the time, and he wanted me to spit in a pot and I couldn't and every time I tried to spit I wanted to be sick. It was really horrible the way he treated me. Because of being in the medical profession I notice things like that as I'm into training doctors and that one was not one of mine. I'm sure no-one told him that this is a victim not a criminal. I'm sure no one said anything to him.

Jenny, whose house had been broken into at 3 a.m. and who had been kept prisoner for several hours, was appalled by the medical examination and the length of time it took:

> The police doctor was the worst person. I was with the police for 12 hours. I think all police doctors should be women. He was most unpleasant. He had a list of things to do that he methodically went through. Some of it was dreadful like unwrapping yourself on pieces of brown paper until you are quite naked. This was followed by a long internal examination. He said he had to remove four pubic hairs, and just pulled them viciously out. I was in a state of hysteria.

Part of the difficulty appears to be the undue concentration on the investigatory aspects to the neglect of humane considerations. The inflexible implementation of procedures may sometimes override common sense and lead to the victim's unnecessary discomfort. One complainant was not allowed to drink for five hours after an horrendous assault, although she had not had oral sex.

Some doctors failed to explain why certain procedures were necessary. In Nora's case, where the assailant had broken into her bedroom, but had not in fact raped her, she said:

> They did the whole bit – spit in the tube and swabs of this and swabs of that. It was all very degrading. He didn't explain what they were doing it for. It's just such an awful experience. It's as simple as that.

Forensic evidence is of course, relevant only in establishing that intercourse took place, not whether it took place with or without consent. However, there is a great deal of fuzzy thinking around this simple statement, and forensic evidence can be used against rather than for the complainant in a number of ways, some of them insidious as the interviews reveal. In the absence of vaginal injuries, which are rare, forensic evidence can be used by the defence to argue that the woman consented. Arguments about whether the woman 'lubricated' are particularly pernicious. One police officer interviewed, who had been on the special course on sexual assault at Hendon Police Training College, insisted quite fallaciously that forensic tests could ascertain from the fluids whether or not the complainant had consented. If some police believe this, it is not surprising that jurors are often confused.

Four of the complainants were examined in rape examination suites but the surroundings were not viewed as the main priority. In the case of the 72 year old, she was examined at home. In the other cases the women were examined in doctor's surgeries. Rape suites were not really appreciated when most women wanted above all else to be examined by a woman doctor, not a man. As Anna explained:

> The police medical centre was absolutely beautiful and they were after spending something like 1.2 million to do it up, but the female doctor wouldn't come out and the only one who would was a man doctor. They did say they would report her (the woman doctor) for not coming out. The doctor who came was a bit pissed off having to get out of bed in the middle of the night. They couldn't get a woman.

She explained how because they couldn't find a woman doctor she had agreed to being examined by a man. She had regretted this afterwards. She explained why:

> I think I was mistaken in doing that because after that I just freaked at the thought of any internal investigations, let alone by a man. I thought it wouldn't make any difference to me whether it was a man or a woman but it did matter a lot. The doctor was business like and not sympathetic.

> Just a few things that stood out to me when I thought about what was happening there. At one point the doctor examining me said 'Well your vagina feels moist, seems like a normal vagina' and I thought 'What is he telling me that for, is he saying I enjoyed it or there is no trauma there so it did not happen?' I did not really know what his comment was for. I was lying on the couch with that paper sheet underneath me and he was pulling out pubic hairs with what looked like automatic tweezers which pull the hair but cut it as well.

Delays in finding a doctor to undertake the examinations was another area of complaint. Some women had to wait for hours while in a state of shock. Women are not allowed to drink or wash, so are often in great discomfort. A further area of concern was the realization that the doctor's report might well be used as evidence. Several women were concerned about the impression they were giving and some perceived the doctor as threatening as Jenny explained:

> You are very sensitive and everything that is said becomes unkind although it may not have been intended. You are so exposed and you know that the reactions and comments of the doctor are going to validate what you've said and his reactions and comments are actually what's happened to you or comments on the state of your body or whatever. I really feel that in shock you tend to be bright and businesslike. I felt I was being too cheery and I wasn't sobbing and I thought 'Is he thinking that it's just a lark or something?' You're just so aware of your own responses but then they are going ahead without you having much control over them, because you've got so much going on inside your head and you're on automatic pilot. So you say 'Yes thank you I'll get on the couch' when really what you want to say is 'Go away, leave me alone I want to go to bed and just forget about it.'

> I know they've got to do it immediately as soon as possible afterwards, but I would have expected the doctor to say a few kind or more personal things. He was very impersonal and very distant. If he would have said – 'You must be feeling bad' or something, but I don't remember him saying anything like that. He did explain what was going to be done in the medical. I just felt that he didn't have any sympathy or compassion and he had no notion of what state I was in. He was just doing his job so that he could go back to bed. I didn't get a good feeling from him, whereas I did from some of the police officers.

Being seen by a woman doctor did not, however, prevent one woman from being very dissatisfied with the questions she was asked. The overall effect of cross-examining women during the medical can lead them to feel they are to blame for the attack. Anything more likely to undermine their confidence, already shaken by the horror of the attack, is difficult to visualize as Fiona, who had been raped by a stranger, explained:

> It was her attitude. It was like it was a big effort that she had been called out at 7 a.m. in the morning. She could have been a lot

more sympathetic in explaining what she was doing. She said she would explain everything when I had had a bath, but when I got back from having my bath she was gone. It was afterwards that I found out why the medical doctor asks questions like 'when was the last time you had sex?' and these questions are brought up in court. As it turned out she said 'how long have you known your boyfriend' and I said 'Well actually he was my childhood sweetheart' and she said 'Alright'. She made me feel like everything was a trap or something and that almost everything would be held against me. Even like the alcohol test they did on me. Although the alcohol test showed up clear there was very low level of alcohol on my breath, I thought they'd use it against me. It seems they're out to get you all the time. I don't know how they'd have gone on about my asking for it [the rape] when I'd never met him before.

### *VD/HIV testing*

Of the survivors in the US 1992 National Women's Study 'Rape in America: A Report to the Nation'[1] 40 per cent said they feared contracting HIV. The question of HIV and sexual assault is only just beginning to be addressed in Britain. It raises all sorts of crucial questions such as whether suspects should under some circumstances be tested. The long delays before trials mean that the victim needs to have access to these results quickly. Clearly in the event of being infected, even if this is unlikely, immediate testing is essential. It is not at present possible to pinpoint the moment or source of infection, but it may soon be possible to match infections with source (see Moran 1994). Some British National Health Service sexual assault counselling agencies are already encountering women who have been found to be HIV-positive after sexual assaults. According to some researchers in the US some women are carrying condoms as a preventive measure, so that in the event of an assault they can try and persuade the assailant to use protection (see Moran 1994).

Complainants in our research experienced particular difficulty in getting VD tests carried out. Several suggested that it would have helped if they had had a piece of paper documenting that they had been raped so that they did not have to announce this often at the admission desk in the clinic in front of other people. This caused great embarrassment as one woman explained:

The next traumatic thing was the clinic. I had been told that there was a time when people who had been raped were specifically able to go and there'd be a nice environment. I walked in and there were men sitting with their girlfriends and when I got to the hatch I had to announce it because the woman behind were looking at me as if to say 'What's the matter with you? I was astounded myself at my own physical reaction to being examined. The doctor had to stop several times during the examination. I wanted to have a thorough examination, even the HIV test because I wanted to know everything. It was a really unpleasant experience, despite the fact that I had a very sympathetic woman. If it had been a man I don't know what I would have done. We had a long chat and talked about everything.

Several women were so traumatized by the medical examination that they could not face going to have a VD test let alone be tested for HIV as Anna, who failed to go to University College Hospital, explained:

I was told to go to hospital to have VD tests, but after the medical examination, I just couldn't do it. I mean that examination was worse than what had happened to me. Basically she used her fingers on me – this nurse who was trying to examine me. I started screaming and shaking and just kept screaming at her to get away from me. I just couldn't cope with it. The porter came out and said 'Oh my God, I'll get another nurse, she's got a smaller hand and she's really gentle'. I've never gone to a doctor since, only ever a female doctor. Even when I gave birth I refused a male surgeon to come in and insisted on a woman.

Mary could not face having an HIV test until two years later:

I actually went for an AIDS test about two years after the attack. I went through a lot of discomfort waiting for the results. I ended up talking to the nurse for about an hour and I was absolutely traumatized by it. I think I just felt that, after the rape, I was worried that I might be pregnant, and then, I wasn't. But I thought this would be another hurdle to go through.

## The need for more women police surgeons (Forensic Medical Examiners)

A number of other studies had indicated that complainants were rarely given the choice of a woman doctor. The Women's National

Commission (1985) reported that in some areas complainants were given a real choice of a male or female surgeon whereas in others they were not. There was clearly still a widespread shortage of women police surgeons. In the Metropolitan Police Division in 1985 only eleven out of 87 police surgeons were women. The report recommended that every woman who had been sexually assaulted should be able to insist on having a woman doctor to examine her. In 1986 when the Home Office issued another circular, the need to recruit more female police surgeons, or to employ more women doctors specifically for the examination, was emphasized. It was recognized that in theory this is offered, but in practice a woman doctor was often not available.

Professor Jennifer Temkin, who carried out a study of the medical treatment of rape victims (Temkin 1996), interviewed twenty-three women who reported rape to the Sussex police from 1991 to 1993. Fourteen of these had been medically examined and were interviewed in depth about their views of the experience. None had been examined in a police station, but only two had been examined in a rape examination suite, two in hospital and the other ten in doctors' surgeries. Additionally, she found that although general practitioners were generally used and a rota system operated, there was still a shortage of female doctors prepared to do forensic work. Police officers reported long delays before victims could be seen by a doctor and sometimes facilities outside the area had to be called on.

The Northumbria REACH (Maddock and Scott 1996) study, discussed in Chapter 6, included giving questionnaires to police officers about their views of the medical services. An alliance between the Tyneside Rape Crisis Centre and the Northumbria police in the early 1980s had led to the recruitment of 35 women doctors who became known as the Women Police Doctors Groups. Male police surgeons did not approve, probably due to the overtime rates paid for night work which they regarded as one of their 'perks'. This has been a problem in other areas. By the mid-1990s the police reported that the doctors list often needed updating. They also complained that the doctor chose where the complainant would be examined and this often involved her having to travel long distances. They considered that easier availability of women doctors would improve the service offered which could be achieved if more doctors participated in the scheme. A number of officers additionally commented on the need for doctors to be up to date with taking samples and forensic packaging.

In Temkin's (1996) study of complainants' reactions to the medical, the findings were generally negative. Twelve (86 per cent) were wholly, mainly or partly negative, so that only two women were entirely positive. Four gave a mixed response and a further four were mainly negative, but made one or two positive comments about the support received during the medical from a female police officer present. Temkin's analysed the responses to cover the following themes: examination by a male doctor, the doctor's manner and attitude, the way in which the examination was conducted and the examination itself.

Nine out of fourteen women were medically examined by a female doctor, considerably more than in our study. Four of the remaining five commented negatively about being examined by a man. Temkin (1996: 17) strongly recommends that 'a sufficient number of fully trained, empathetic, female doctors to examine complainants more or less as soon as they report the offence should be a minimum requirement for an efficient consumer-led service for victims'. She adds that this is not the only reform which is needed, but that some of the procedures should be dropped as they are not forensically necessary. The plucking of pubic hairs was a case in point. The practice was discontinued by the Metropolitan Police Forensic Science Laboratory in 1990 after requests by doctors who pointed out that later blood tests could provide such information where it was needed.

Another issue Temkin raises is how much questioning of the victim by the doctor is actually necessary. Victims are usually made to repeat their statement although the information could easily be obtained from the police officer. There are two further problems that can arise from the doctor taking too many details. Firstly, defence lawyers make much of any discrepancies between different accounts, and, even more unfairly, on some occasions glean details of the past sexual history of the victim which they confront her with in court. In a rape case which was monitored by Lees (1997a) at the Central Criminal Court the fact that the complainant had had an abortion (totally disconnected from the alleged rape), was used with great effect to discredit her in court. It is, therefore, vital that the doctor does not include such details in the medical report in order to avoid its use by the defence. A second consideration is that there is evidence that the complainant's statements and medical reports are circulated in prison as pornography (see Radford 1989). Temkin concludes that distress occasioned to rape victims by medical examinations has yet to be minimized. She persuasively (1996: 18) argues that women in the 1990s describe the medical in such terms as: ' "more degrading and demoralising than the rape itself", "a nightmare", "another violation", "being raped all over again" which comprises a very serious and disappointing indictment of the progress which has been achieved in the provision of criminal justice for victims of rape'.

Similar findings emerged from interviews with eight women undertaken by Victim Support (January 1996).[2] Two women who were seen in a rape examination suite and given relevant information by a woman doctor were very satisfied with their treatment. They described the doctors as 'brilliant' (ibid. 20) and 'wonderful' (ibid. 37). One of these women movingly described what happened: 'I walked into the room and this lady came straight up to me and said "Oh my God, what has he done to you?" It was wonderful. I wish everyone could have had her. How could they ever use male doctors?' (Even in this case the victim was not given all the medical information about her condition – she was not told, for example that she had internal cuts until the court case.)

The other women reported that they were too often given no real choice, as they were only able to see a doctor if they were prepared to wait for long periods of time. One woman, for example, was told she could see a male doctor straight away, but if she wanted to see a female doctor she would have to wait all evening.

Three women were not even given the choice nor were they seen in a rape examination suite. One of these specifically asked for a woman doctor but was told that none was available. Another, not given the choice, commented: 'I was seen by a man doctor who was quite old and I felt uncomfortable with him. I would have preferred a woman but no-one asked me'. She was provided with no advice on medical matters. Instead she had to find the information out for herself (ibid. 27). One woman described the examination as 'horrendous' and said she definitely would not have gone through with reporting it if she had known what the medical would be like. The report commented that a sympathetic female doctor in a specially designed rape examination suite would make all the difference to what was essentially a traumatic experience and recommended the urgent recruitment of more female doctors who should be given specialist training. It specified that the examination should take place without delay and that every woman should have ready access to specially prepared facilities for the medical.

When interviewed in January 1993, one Forensic Medical Examiner told us that there was a chronic shortage of women surgeons. Part of the difficulty she attributed to male surgeon's inability to appreciate that there was a need to restrict this work to female doctors and anxiety that they would be missing out. While appreciating the need to give victims a choice, some of the male doctors accused the police of persuading women to ask for a female doctor. Forensic medical work is very high pressure demanding work and the hours are unsociable, which adds to the difficulties of recruiting women. Women also may be more reluctant to give evidence in court which they may regard as an ordeal.

It appears that in some areas real progress is being made. In the REACH study where a voluntary Woman Doctors' Scheme had been set up and adequately funded, 46 women who had been medically examined filled in a questionnaire about the experience. The majority of women expressed high levels of satisfaction with the service. One woman wrote 'the police who dealt with my case were very caring and understanding and totally abolished all the thoughts I had on the way women were treated in rape cases' (Maddock and Scott 1995: 4).

What is of crucial importance is that police officers and forensic doctors are aware of the research into the effects of rape and the extreme vulnerability of complainants. Koss and Harvey (1988: 166), American psychologists who investigated medical examinations in the US, have some relevant suggestions to make about how doctors should behave. A few understanding words can make all the difference to the woman's experience. They suggested several helpful expressions that should be memorized for use with victims of sexual assault such as: (a) I am so sorry this happened to you; (b) You're safe now; (c) No matter what you did, you did not deserve to be a victim of a crime; and (d) I know you handled the situation right because you're alive. The problem with this approach is that if doctors have to memorize statements such as these rather than behaving spontaneously, they could well still say the wrong thing. It could also be argued that memorizing phrases suggests inadequate training

It is also vital that forensic doctors become more aware of the reasons for excluding information from the medical report about the complainant's past sexual history unless it is strictly relevant to the rape. The Forensic Medical Examiner we interviewed said she had been to court hundreds of times and previous sexual history still seems to come out, although it is not supposed to be relevant. She also commented that defence lawyers do pursue a hostile line of questioning when cross-examining doctors, but that doctors can handle it. This may be true of her but certainly is not true of all doctors.

The significance of a sympathetic hearing to the complainant's recovery has been well documented. In her study of the aftermath of rape, Cathy Roberts (1989), a founder member of the London Rape Crisis Centre, indicated how much difference a clear, supportive and positive response could make to a woman's self image, and to the way she views her experiences. The importance of other people's reactions and the attitude of society should not be underestimated. In her study of the records of thirty women who contacted a rape crisis centre, she found that during the year following the attack, a third showed signs of depression, and had some kind of sexually transmitted disease, pregnancy or injuries to cope with, and many experienced feelings of guilt. In coping with rape, Roberts argued, women were actually coping with a social definition and reaction to rape and to victims.

## Interviewees' views of Victim Support and Rape Crisis

There are two main organizations that aim to provide some kind of counselling for the survivors of sexual assault. Rape Crisis is predominantly a telephone help line set up by rape survivors and providing some counselling, mainly over the telephone. The roots of rape crisis work lie in the recognition that sexual violence is widely experienced by women and results from women's unequal position in society. Centres developed from the consciousness raising groups of the 1970s Women's Liberation Movement, where validating women's experiences was seen as leading to direct action for social change. Speaking out was seen as a necessary first step to raising the issue as a political issue, since women suffered in silence, often blaming themselves. Central to the position of many of these groups was a political aim of transforming the relations between men and women and shifting the responsibility for violence from women onto men. In some centres all the volunteers had to have experienced sexual assault themselves.

Rape Crisis work in the US and Britain was faced with contradictions between the need for funding and the problems of collective leadership. In the early days there was resistance to any kind of bureaucratic hierarchical managerial organization and all decisions were taken collectively. This along with a strong emphasis on confidentiality often conflicted with the requirements of funding authorities and was clearly an important factor behind the withdrawal of funds from the London Rape Crisis centre which occurred around the time of our field work.

By the mid-1990s there were about seventy centres in England and Wales, each working autonomously and many registered as charities. Some employed staff while others struggled on very minimal amounts. In order to counteract the isolation and underfunding of centres, in October 1996 a Federation of Rape Crisis Centres was launched in Manchester[3] to provide central co-ordination and develop a more professional approach. It also aimed to provide a forum for debate within the movement, uniform training, and better monitoring standards of practice for services. Many of the centres have changed their name and taken on a more social services therapeutic approach, where the political aim of challenging male violence is no longer so prominent. Even so, funds are increasingly being channelled into Victim Support which means that rape crisis centres are providing only a skeletal service or facing closure.

Rape Crisis has also been hit by cuts in local government spending even when its structure had been adapted to the stipulations of the funding bodies. This means that very few provide face to face counselling, and in London one telephone line which only operates for a few hours a day was functioning when we undertook our research. This was reflected in such comments from our interviewees as:

> I had extreme difficulty finding support services. Every time I rang rape crisis over a period of a week, their phone was engaged. I ultimately received counselling but I had to pay for it.

Victim Support is a nationwide and more politically palatable service, partly funded by the Home Office, which provides help to all victims of crime. It secured Home Office funding when, in the 1980s, government ideology and financial uncertainly were leading in other areas of public service to a curtailment of service delivery and a reduced level of state involvement. A national charity, it represented a voluntary response emphasizing individuals helping other individuals from within their community. It avoided political involvement and successfully gained the support of the police and the Home Office. By 1990 there were over 300 victim support schemes in the country (Mawby and Walklate 1994) and this had risen to 378 by 1996 (Victim Support 1996).

Unlike Rape Crisis, Victim Support does not specialize in sexual assault cases, but it is developing some expertise in the area. Following a working party report in 1985 on how the service should develop, the first national training programme for work with women who had suffered sexual violence was published (Victim Support 1987) and between 1991 and 1996, the number of women referred to the scheme following a rape or sexual assault doubled. In 1995 Victim Support schemes offered a service to over 15,400 victims of rape and other sexual offences (Victim Support 1996). Some women are put in touch with Victim Support by the police, but increasingly women get in contact themselves. In 1995 almost a third of the women offered help, some of whom had not reported the assault to the police, made direct contact with their local scheme.

In Islington, Victim Support had developed good liaison with the local police and all cases of sexual assault were referred to them. Victim Support would then write a letter offering their services. In fact one of the paid workers had herself worked for Rape Crisis as a paid worker. There has been a particular focus on providing counselling for the survivors of rape and sexual assault and training was regularly provided by professional counsellors. In 1992 some face-to-face counselling was provided by counselling services in the borough. On the whole, the feedback from complainants living in Islington was positive, although some women would have liked more intensive counselling than was available at the time. Some cases are referred on to the Woman's Therapy Centre, an independent service which is fee paying. Two of the complainants, who had received compensation, had spent some of it on counselling.

However, some of the complainants interviewed did not live in Islington and had therefore been contacted by their local Victim Support Service. Two of these said they had not been told about Victim Support. Sylvia said:

> I think the police could have said that Victim Support was available and that way you could have the opportunity to decide if you wanted to go to them or not. Perhaps they could even put you in touch with someone in your local area and not necessarily in the area where the assault happened.

Jacky said 'They didn't offer me no Victim Support. No, they didn't offer me nothing'. Ann regretted not being informed of Rape Crisis:

> I thought it was wrong that you didn't get a choice whether you wanted to go to Victim Support or the Rape Crisis Centre. I don't know whether Rape Crisis would have been any different. I think talking to someone who has been through it would have been much easier instead of having to explain everything as you go along. They did keep me informed though which was good.

Many of the women in Islington found Victim Support invaluable. Lizzie, who had suffered an extremely violent attack said:

> I did see the woman from Victim Support who told me all about the court case and what to expect. She was great and said the court case wouldn't be easy so she really prepared me. And she actually came with me.

Fiona, who had been raped, would have preferred to go to Rape Crisis:

Victim Support were good but they are there for everything; like burglaries, mugging etc. whereas Rape Crisis would be more specialized. They did give me a Victim Support number at work and then the doctor suggested it to me afterwards and I rang them up and I spoke to somebody on the phone but to be quite honest it was a dead loss. It was stupid, it's like talking to somebody and saying yeah, yeah, yeah....Because it's part of the counsellor's job to just talk. But you feel like when you're talking to them that they don't really understand what you're going through. I've spoke to other girls who've been through the same kind of thing and they feel the same way. You feel like you're talking to a brick wall. If you've got someone who says yeah I do know I've been through it and you know they've been through it by what they tell you, you feel better. I just spoke to them one night and then didn't bother.

Carolyn, who lived in Tottenham, was not impressed with Victim Support, and had found the worker patronizing:

Maybe she was understaffed but she was very strange. I was feeling very awkward about it and she kept going on about my girls and she just made me feel like a real victim who might have just come out of care or an orphanage. It was something about her attitude that didn't make me feel any stronger. It made me feel delinquent. She kept saying things like 'A lot of people say that people ask for it', but sometimes I think that people who state things like that, in some way they really believe it. It's like when someone says 'I don't doubt your word'; it makes you wonder if they really do doubt it. The police never once made such a statement. Anyway she never showed up for the court case which was just as well. It was odd...but I would have liked to be able to talk to someone about it.

Nora, whose horrific ordeal has already been described, suffered long-term effects, exacerbated, no doubt, by her husband's death. She found Victim Support helpful, but was clearly in need of long-term counselling. This is how she describes her predicament over three years after the attack:

I only saw the woman from Victim Support for a couple of weeks. I didn't really take it seriously to begin with. She was a lovely person, really nice but I think it's something people can't help you with. I've still got the horrors now at night, almost every night when I go to sleep. I don't go to sleep till 5 o'clock in the morning. When I do go to sleep this thing re-enacts in my mind. Sometimes I get a couple of nights free but it invariably starts again. It's a horrible feeling because I get all the fears. I think I'm going to have a heart attack but what can you do, nobody can do anything for you. There is nothing worse than going to bed knowing you're going to get these horrors of a night. It's a terrible thing and it petrifies me.

She describes how when she went to her doctor over a year later, he was no help:

I asked the doctor to put me on something stronger than Nurofen but he says I couldn't afford it as he couldn't give me anything else on prescription. If you go private and pay you can have what you want but not with the health service.

Here there is clearly a need for long-term counselling and victims of serious assaults should be told about the long-term effects and where they can get help (see Newburn 1993). At present such help is only available in some areas and for limited periods. The Avon Sexual Assault Centre in Bristol offers long-term counselling to victims of sexual assault, and is funded by the local authority.

The demand for counselling services more geared to intensive work came out clearly in the interviews. Victim Support services vary from area to area and the volunteers are often not experienced in this specialist area of counselling. Rape Crisis is very underfunded and only operates a telephone line; little else is available. Here are some women's experiences of seeking help:

I phoned the Samaritans and wouldn't recommend it to anybody. The first time I phoned them I got this bloke who was actually quite sympathetic but who sort of paused and I wondered what happened and then he said 'I'm sorry but perhaps you could phone back tomorrow'. I phoned back the next day and spoke to a woman who said 'Well what's your problem?' And I said 'I've been raped' and she said 'Yes and what exactly is your problem with it? What is it that you cannot deal with?' I just found it totally horrific. It was terrible that you couldn't speak to anyone about it.

One woman was referred by the police surgeon for counselling:

The surgeon also referred me to a therapist who they'd had an arrangement with. I went to a therapist for about a year. I started going once a week and then whenever I could. She kept me going really and my life revolved around going to see her. I paid when I could until I gave up my job and then when I got pregnant I did not pay at all.

Lizzie, was one of several women who did not feel they needed any help at the time, but then had a delayed reaction. Fortunately in this case, she had the help of a sympathetic doctor:

They sent a psychiatric nurse round to see me but I was determined to say that everything was all right. It was not until a year later that everything started to come out. I went to the doctor for something completely different and when he asked if I was all right, I just burst into tears and we had a long talk about it. He put me in touch with the Woman's Therapy Centre and I went on a group therapy weekend. We all felt it was too short so we kept in touch and actually held sessions at each other's houses which was really good.

The other need is for self-defence courses to be run in all areas. Several women spoke of the value of having been to such courses. Liz, who had fought off her attacker by first talking to him and then moving when he slightly released his grip, said:

I had been to self-defence classes a couple of weeks before and talking had been mentioned. I told him I was two months pregnant and my husband was waiting for me upstairs.

The extent to which self-defence worked depended a lot on the circumstances.

In terms of the physical aspect, classes didn't help because he was a lot taller than me and kicking him didn't help. The self-defence classes tell you to do certain things in certain circumstances but in reality it happens so fast and it doesn't work out the way the classes instruct you. But I did get away.

Sharon had been thrown to the ground and when the man had kissed her she had bitten his tongue:

One minute I was pressing the button for the lift and the next thing I was on the floor and he was on top of me and tearing my clothes off. I bit him and he got off me and ran. It was not a conscious decision. I just did it. I was completely shocked as well. I couldn't breathe. I kept thinking I was going to throw up.

## Complainants' views of court

Both police and victims complained of the appalling inadequacies of court facilities where there was often no heating, bare furnishing and poor canteen facilities. If the defendant was on bail the complainant and the defendant often had to wait in the same room. Frequently, the complainant had no idea what would happen. The experience of Tina who had been indecently assaulted, thrown on the ground and later threatened with retaliation if she went ahead with the court case was traumatic:

> I had no preparation. At the time of the court he was there. They called me in. He kept saying he fell over. My cousin was going back to Ireland. She was being threatened. She was having bottles thrown at her. She was being threatened by this bloke's friends. I told them about it.

Sharing a waiting room and canteen facilities with the suspect understandably unnerved a number of complainants:

> I think you should be warned that you are going to have to share the canteen facilities in the court with defendants. I wasn't as scared by the experience as some women, but seeing him was strange. I tend to take a lot out on myself. I'm sure you could get really scared in this situation

Another woman echoed this:

> I would have liked not to have to sit where he had to sit. I don't see why I had to sit in the same room. It's the same kind of personal space invasion so the perpetrator should have to sit in a separate room. I've never seen him since thank goodness. I'm not sure what I would do if I saw him again.

Like Brenda, a highly successful professional woman who experienced a minor indecent assault also found the court unnerving:

What was interesting was the subjective experience of being in court and seeing the person there, and also feeling that he was very close to home. I didn't know what he was capable of doing in retaliation. For all I knew he could have been drunk or a thug.

I think the court was awful. It was a disaster. Firstly I was really quite frightened of bumping into him (the defendant). There's no separate waiting area at Highbury and when I arrived I was frightened that when I got into the lift, he might be in the lift as well...Then when I was giving evidence, I mumbled because I was nervous and the Court Clerk kept telling me to speak up so I was really frightened and nervous and worried. His defence was saying 'Wasn't I just a hysterical woman' and I was saying 'No I'm not hysterical'. The only person who was encouraging was the magistrate who was smiling encouraging me. Then when the defendant gave evidence he mumbled and I couldn't hear anything. The reason he was allowed to mumble was that it appeared it was my evidence which was the basis of the trial. In rape cases you shouldn't end up being torn to shreds. They shouldn't have made me speak loudly and slowly and then me not being able to hear what he said very well. That's because I'm a witness. I'm not really part of this. I mean it's all about me but I'm not part of it.

Women are still asked to give their address to the court, a procedure which seems to be at odds with the legal requirement that the anonymity of victims should be protected. It represents a denial of the threat the woman feels after an attack: 'They shouldn't make you give your address because he didn't know my address before'.

Even complainants who had been quite randomly attacked were very aware that they might well be blamed for some kind of provocation, for example by wearing particular clothes. Brenda thought she might have been treated differently if she had not been respectably dressed:

I was walking down the road with my daughter. In a way having my daughter helped. The thing is if I had been wearing a very low cut top with a mini skirt, that doesn't matter. It's not an invitation for people to do things that you don't agree to or consent, but as it was I was wearing something more covered up and had my 11-year-old daughter with me. I am a respectable sort of person not a tart. I think it would have been different if I had turned up in those sort of clothes.

Nora, whose experience with the police had been so unfortunate, found going to court a gruelling experience. The fact that the case came up when her husband's cancer had progressed, just after he had had a brain operation, could not have helped. He was too ill to go to court. Nora could not understand why she was bombarded with questions:

> The defence said 'I'm not saying you're lying but I suggest you were dreaming and you dreamt this'. I said 'I suggest you're a bloody fool if you think that I would stand here and say all this if it's not true'. I just thought 'Stand down you bloody fool'. (The judge questioned the defence lawyer about her line of questioning.) It's horrible because your mouth goes dry and you walk into that court and they've all got wigs on and it's awful really. I thought I was going to drop. I must have a strong heart not to have had a heart attack from all this. When I get night terrors I think I'm going to get a heart attack.

Although the assailant was sentenced to eight years imprisonment, Nora was worried that he might return on his release.

> I think sometimes about him coming back when he gets out. That worries me. I would like to know when he is released on parole. I heard that no sooner are they in prison than they are released on parole.

Carolyn had this to add:

> I think a screen would really have helped. I really do. When I left I just burst into tears and I felt I hadn't done very well and that I'd ruined it, but the police said I had done fine.

Una, raped by her estranged husband, asked during the interview whether she had any preparation for the court, replied:

> Well you can't prepare for that. They did try to prepare me, but the formality of it, you can't be prepared for that especially in the Crown Court. It's not so bad in the magistrates' court. I thought I could handle it but the onslaught was so bad, and to me going to court and the papers afterwards was the worst thing, The attack itself was bad but there was nothing I could do about that. I was pleased I did it still.

She described the stress of the long delay before the case came to court and what it was like going to court:

> Going to court was the most traumatic experience of my life. The build up nearly made me drop the charges. The people from the Domestic Violence Unit were going to come but something came up and they couldn't. The court was horrendous. The cross-examination was awful. I just broke down. The whole manipulations was awful. After, the local newspaper wrote an awful spread about him getting off. I lived locally and then they printed that. I should have gone to the press council and done all sorts of things but I just wanted to forget about it all. I did phone the *Gazette* and questioned them about how twisted the story was.

She described how the slowness of the court procedure was also a problem:

> The whole thing was just horrendous and it took a year of my life. It was just complete turmoil. I was lucky because I had property and a good job as a manager. Most women lack security. I think if cases got to court quicker a lot more charges would go to court. After several months it fades and you start thinking that you don't want to go through with it, especially if you have kids. The kids were used as pawns and they really went through it. That's why I nearly dropped the charges.

Since this research was undertaken the Victim Support, Crown Court witness service has been introduced, and since April 1996 has been operating in every Crown Court centre in England and Wales. It offers information and support to victims, witnesses and their families before, during and after the trial. It can arrange familiarization visits to show witnesses around an empty court room before the trial. Volunteers provide information and explanation about court procedures and can accompany witnesses into court when they are called to give evidence. It also provides private waiting areas in the court to ensure that victims and witnesses do not have to sit near the defendant or his or her family (see Victim Support 1996: 4).

The Victim Support (1996) survey of witness services found that there were four main areas of concern: the cross-examination, lack of protection, waiting times in court and changes of trial dates. It recommended that practical arrangements still needed to be made to avoid contact between the defendant and the complainant and to provide support prior to the court case; that the defendant should be removed from court while the witness enters and leaves; that her address should not be read out in court; and the use of screens should be allowed.

## Use of forensic evidence in court

Anna Clark (1987), a historian, argues that the detail women are required to go into to describe the assault has increased with the development of forensic science. Forensic doctors do indeed play a crucial 'expert' role in analysing women's responses and sometimes give uninformed and distorting accounts of the 'typical' bodily signs and symptoms of rape victims. This can mean that the jury is misled by inaccurate and false accounts which can seriously contribute to false acquittals. Lees (1997a), in her monitoring of trials at the Central Criminal Court, came across a number of cases where medical examinations had been used by the defence to imply that the complainant was making a false allegation. Since the defence counsel can call his/her own doctor (and pay him/her a fee) to question the evidence of the police doctor, it is all too easy for them to make such insinuations.

The complainant's distress is not seen as corroborative in English and Welsh law (although, paradoxically, it is in Scottish law). However, the absence of distress can be used against her. For example Judge Williams, in summing up the Diggle case on 20 August 1993, argued that the woman's distress cannot corroborate other evidence but can confirm it:

> What is not independent is Ms H's apparent distress when she ran into her friend's bedroom. Nor is it when the policewoman asked her about what had happened as it is not an independent source, although it is not irrelevant. It may show her conduct after the alleged incident. It may confirm the other evidence.

One difficulty jurors experience is that rape often has no visible signs. This is why asking the victim about the aftermath of rape is so vital. In the Vicarage rape case, Michael Saward, whose daughter was savagely raped by several men, admitted that he misread his daughter's inward state by her outward demeanour. When interviewed on television (Everyman 1990) he said: 'Both the judge and myself made, I suppose you might say, a masculine response'. This may well be true, but why, then, is the complainant not asked about her reaction? 'What are we meant to do?' Jill Saward asks, 'Wear a Sign? Nobody in the court ever asked how I felt, or asked anybody else how I was' (Everyman 1990).

In another case, on 1 September 1993 at the Old Bailey, Judge Smedley commented on why evidence of the complainant's distress should not be regarded as relevant at all:

> A word of warning. If the account the complainant is giving was completely fabricated, you may think she is clever, then clever enough to act out distress.

A common tactic used by the defence to support the idea of a woman making a false allegation, is to suggest that the complainant's reactions are not typical of a rape victim. The prosecution rarely inform the jury that there is no simple 'typical' reaction. For many the reaction is delayed. Some women express anxiety immediately; others remain calm.

In a trial monitored by Lees (1997a) of a man separately tried for raping five women, in which he was acquitted of raping four of them, evidence in one trial that the complainant had not broken down was used to imply that she was making it up. In her cross-examination the defence counsel argued that Jessica was 'not distressed at all' and had cried for only twenty seconds while talking but had then smiled and carried on talking. The defence counsel then cross-examined her in the following terms:

DEFENCE COUNSEL: So the doctor has got it wrong?

JESSICA: Well, I was distressed.

DEFENCE COUNSEL: Were you showing...the doctor can probably only go on what she can see. Did you show any signs of distress to the doctor beyond the 20 seconds?

JESSICA: Well, for a while I did, yeah, but I was calm as well.

DEFENCE COUNSEL: What signs, in the light of his Honour's questions, were you showing of distress to this doctor?

JESSICA: Well, I did cry and...

DEFENCE COUNSEL: Anything else? I mean, is this doctor right or wrong or just mistaken?

JESSICA: Well maybe, I wasn't showing signs of distress at some times, but I was feeling it.

DEFENCE COUNSEL: I see. So this doctor – it was a woman doctor – failed to see that underneath it you were, in fact, distressed and, as you said, you were not at all distressed, making the point you cried for about 20 seconds, but then smiled and carried on talking. What is the picture that we should have?

JESSICA: I was distressed, but she was doing her best to try and, you know, be nice and cheer me up.

As Jessica explained:

> A lot of people expect you to be in tears because that sort of thing happened, but I'm not that sort of person. I don't show anyone my feelings. What happened to me, I deal with it in my own way. I don't need anyone else's help.

Jessica is perfectly right and the judge should know about the research findings in regard to the rape trauma syndrome rather than collude with the defence counsel's position.

On only one occasion in Lees's research did a forensic doctor refute the defence counsel's suggestion that anger was an unusual response to rape and that more typically, victims reacted with tears. Her emphasis that women can respond in different ways, that a moist vulva does not indicate consent, and that rape does not necessarily leave any visible signs of damage or reddening, was crucial in leading to the conviction of the defendant.

DEFENCE COUNSEL: What state was she in?
DOCTOR: She seemed very annoyed.
DEFENCE COUNSEL: Would you expect to see that in a rape victim?
DOCTOR: You see all sorts of reactions.
DEFENCE COUNSEL: You don't usually see annoyance or anger.
DOCTOR: Oh yes you do.
DEFENCE COUNSEL: Her vulva was moist. Do you attach any significance to that?
DOCTOR: Moisture could be consistent with sucking.
DEFENCE COUNSEL: Can you help me with this? If a woman is being subjected to forceful intercourse at a time when she describes herself as rigid, wouldn't you expect to see reddening?
DOCTOR: No. Very often you see nothing.

Williams and Holmes (1981) found that about two-thirds of their sample of rape victims expressed feelings of anger towards their assailant and such feelings tended to persist over considerable periods of time (see Newburn 1993).

Lack of injuries too can be taken as indication of consent. In one case lack of supportive proof in the form of material injuries resulting from the woman's resistance was taken as evidence that the woman had consented, even though she claimed she did not and had been frozen with fear.

In rape trials, jurors have been instructed that under the influence of sex women lie so convincingly that they will not only fabricate a story of rape, for example, to avoid being honest with their partner, but to substantiate it they will run naked into the street, cry compulsively, spend the night in a police station, change their name or even move home. The judge does not draw the jury's attention to the fact that most women who have been raped cannot face the ordeal they will have to go through if they complain to the police (many, indeed, cannot face telling anyone); and that they are often threatened with retaliation if they do go to the police. One woman when asked why she had not gone at once to the police replied 'Because he told me that if I told anyone or went to the police, he'd come back for me and the children'. It seems that only if she is half dead can the jury be sure she is not a malicious schemer.

In another case it was implied that because there were no vaginal injuries rape could not have occurred, although bruising is not a typical sign of rape. This is not unusual. In a recent case at Isleworth Crown Court where a persistent sexual offender had been acquitted, the victim ran after the jury and asked them why they had not found him guilty. The jury members told her that they had expected there to be forensic evidence of injuries. Inspector Carol Bristow of Acton Police, when interviewed, said she thought judges and barristers showed a great lack of understanding about this type of offence.

Another young woman, a virgin, whose heart rate and blood pressure were so high according to the examining doctor that 'if the pulse rate went any higher there would have been some kind of heart failure', was deemed by the defence doctor to have developed these symptoms as a result of making a false allegation rather than as a result of the rape!

The medical examination should surely not be used in this way to distort the evidence, but instead juries should be told about the research which has indicated how complainants commonly react to rape.

## Sentencing and criminal injuries compensation

For women who have endured the ordeals described in this report, low sentences, particularly fines and compensation, make a mockery of the whole procedure. Cases that went to magistrates' courts often resulted in fines. Complainants were very ambivalent about accepting money from the defendant, often regarding it as some meagre payment for services rendered under force, something akin to prostitution or 'dirty money'. Other women took a different view but even their comments indicated a certain ambivalence as suggested by Sara's response:

I didn't think about the compensation very much. I suppose I saw the £75 if you like as a reward for having gone to court, for giving information. I didn't see it as payment for touching my breasts.

Tina, whose cousin was threatened with violence if she gave evidence, received little satisfaction from her court appearance. The magistrates did not appear to take the offence seriously.

They called him a molester and everything. They fined him £25 compensation which to this day I haven't got. It's not the money. I just wanted him to suffer the same as I did. I couldn't care less about the money. If you look at what some people get for driving offences. It's bad. So that was the end of it. It was sexual assault. In the paper it was down as sexual assault but all he got was a ticking off and he was told to give me £25. What do I want £25 for? I mean what's that going to compensate me for? I just wanted to see him suffer for what he'd done to me.

The irrelevance of a fine is reiterated by Tina, who was indecently assaulted, and raises the question as to what sexual assault is all about:

I think sexual assault is either about power or about being sick. I've got no idea why he did it. I don't suppose he knows why he did it either. But the court does not make him confront any of the issues at all. I mean he can just walk around all day. Okay there is a bit of a financial penalty but it's not a deterrent really. Nor will it deter people from doing it again. If he could be made to understand why he did it and what effect it has on people he might not do it again.

Many women also expressed anxiety about claiming compensation. Amanda, although she had a degree in English, found she just could not bring herself to write down the details of the attack. She managed to fill out the formalities but just could not explain in her own words what had happened. She had kept the form for a very long time, and kept trying to fill it in but was simply unable to. She finally decided it was just not worth the anxiety.

Women who had been interviewed by the Criminal Injuries Compensation Board often found this a gruelling experience. One woman in the Victim Support study found it the most upsetting experience of the whole ordeal. It takes far too long to claim compensation

which makes it harder for women to get on with their lives as Sandra
explained

> They said they wanted to help me with the compensation. I really
> should go back soon and get that form filled out. I know I have to,
> a couple of stiff drinks and sit me down with a biro. It would take
> about a year and a half to come through anyway. I mean I could
> then put a deposit on a place over in Ireland, my mum and dad
> think by now I should have that all straightened out. So I can say
> right, that's finished, forget about it now completely. 'Cause you
> still think about it. It's not an obsession or anything like that. I
> mean now and again it would just come back.

Sometimes the amount of compensation is insulting. Nora questioned
the meaning of compensation and the amount:

> I did get compensation which I thought was lousy and my
> husband's compensation went back because he had died by the
> time they came round to paying it. I got a thousand pounds which
> I thought was terrible. I wouldn't have known about it but the
> Victim Support lady put me in for it. I suppose when they put a
> price on you and you get that – it's terrible. I had cuts on my arms
> and face and I didn't notice at first that he had cut my arms as
> well.

What to spend the compensation on is an important consideration.
Many women spent it on therapy or counselling or taking taxis.

The Victim Support (1996) study found that six of the eleven
women they interviewed were still waiting for their claims to be
processed, some over two years after the offence took place. One of the
women described the Criminal Injuries Compensation hearing as the
most distressing aspect resulting from reporting the rape. In her case,
the hearing took place in front of a panel which was never shown the
report of the police surgeon. They were not therefore aware of the
evidence backing up her allegation and she was not allowed to see the
police report. The hearing lasted several hours and her claim was
rejected.

Since April 1996, although the amount of money that can be
claimed has been reduced, attempts have been made to improve the
effectiveness of the scheme. Under the Criminal Injuries
Compensation Act 1995 panel members must receive victim awareness
training and under the new tariff system appeal procedures should be

explained to all applicants. It aims to be quicker to administer.

## Conclusion

For over ten years now research has clearly indicated the importance of the availability of women doctors to undertake the medical examination in rape suites that are well equipped and well maintained. These two essential requirements are still not available in all areas.

In 1997 after a long campaign forensic doctors in the Met. can now be paid a retainer. Previously they have only been paid for the examination itself, which has led to doctors insisting that victims should come to their surgeries. With the concentration of resources, complainants may still have to travel some distance, but the advantages of a well equipped centre, where women doctors would always be available, would seem to outweigh the disadvantages.

The use of forensic evidence in court by defence lawyers should be monitored to prevent the presentation of distorted evidence. Again the need to train forensic doctors in post-traumatic stress disorder and rape crisis syndrome is of paramount importance.

This research also indicates that there is a need for adequate long-term counselling to be made available in all areas. Victim Support and Rape Crisis are still under-resourced and long-term counselling is in scarce supply.

# 8 Conclusion

Despite greater official acknowledgement of the serious and persistent nature of sexual and domestic violence reflected in government pronouncements, police force orders and a few legislative reforms, the overall picture to emerge from this book is that very little has changed. Since the setting up of the CPS in 1986, an even lower proportion of assailants in cases of rape and sexual assault has been convicted. This parallels the failure of domestic violence legislation to have any marked effect, leaving the conviction rate of reported domestic assaults at a mere 4 per cent (Channel 4, *Dispatches* 1998). Our own research has covered the full spectrum of rape and sexual assault cases, encompassing attacks by strangers, acquaintances and intimates; attacks in public places and within the domestic domain; 'one-off' assaults and repeat victimization. The evidence leads us to conclude that it is unhelpful and damaging to make a sharp distinction between the classic stranger rape and attacks by men known to their victims. Such a division is spurious, as we know that men who attack strangers can also attack acquaintances and lovers and vice versa (Lees 1997a); it both trivializes the harm caused by all abuses of male power and leaves an ever increasing proportion of complainants – women, children and men – vulnerable to further violence with no effective remedy.

It often seems quite arbitrary whether a case is categorized as rape or assault and in the case of assault the charge can vary from common assault, through ABH to attempted murder (see for example the case of Una recounted in Chapter 3). In marital rape cases, there is often evidence of strangulation, with the victim in some cases losing consciousness (Lees 1997b); these cases could equally well have been classified as attempted murder. A significant proportion of women who have experienced physical assault or threats also report rape. In Kelly's analysis of women who had experienced abuse on more than one occasion 45 per cent had been raped (Kelly *et al.* 1998). Women who have left their husbands or lovers may be harassed, raped or even killed by these men; it is the rejection which often precipitates the violent reaction. This is vividly demonstrated in a case reported in January 1998. A serial rapist on parole from a twelve year prison sentence started a relationship with an accountant whom he met in a nightclub. On being informed by the prison authorities of his record, she ended the relationship but was then harassed by him; finally he raped and then drowned her (Boggan and Marks 1998).

The main barrier to change rests in our view with the apparent intransigence of both police and judicial culture, where the prioritiza-tion of white heterosexual male right continues to reign supreme. In this final chapter, we will assess the possibilities for breaking through this barrier by examining two key issues: first, changes in the composi-tion and culture of the criminal justice system and second, current proposals for reforming the law on rape. Here we will draw on experi-ences in other countries, where some of the reforms that feminists have campaigned for in Britain have already been introduced, with mixed results.

## Spotlight on the Criminal Justice System

### *Police force or police service?*

During the past two decades, British police forces have been on the receiving end of a constant bombardment of criticism, advice and instruction from various quarters. An avalanche of reports and new legislation has created a cumulative pressure for change from a service which, in many ways, still carries the hallmark of its origins in the nineteenth century. It has responded somewhat sluggishly and patchily to these initiatives and has managed to resist some of them altogether. Contradictory messages from central government have sometimes made it difficult for senior officers to know which way to turn. On the one hand, the Conservative government's prioritization of law and order issues throughout the 1980s and 1990s led to a substantial increase in police powers and, at the beginning of this period, a marked improvement in pay and status. On the other hand, the police service, along with the rest of the public sector, has been required to respond to the disciplines of the market. There has also been a shift of power to the centre, so that while still maintaining a degree of autonomy, chief constables have come under increasing scrutiny from government. It is the Home Secretary who now sets national policing objectives and performance indicators for the police, requiring chief constables to produce policing plans consistent with these objectives (see Police and Magistrates' Courts Act 1994).

The imposition of a business ethos and a management style imported from the private sector has in itself proved contradictory. The creation of quality assurance mechanisms and user groups has helped to focus attention on service delivery to members of the public. At the same time, there has been an attempt to separate out the 'core' functions of policing from the more 'peripheral' tasks. The Conservative government believed that 'fighting crime should be the priority for police officers' (Home Office 1993b) and this approach has been endorsed by the Audit Commission, which also favours the restriction of policing to core 'crime fighting' tasks and the hiving off of so-called service or caring functions. As a mere 20 per cent of police time is devoted to explicitly crime control functions, such an approach has serious resource implications for police forces. As Leishman *et al.* (1996) comment: 'Reclaiming the "rubbish" of social service (and other) functions frequently dismissed by the police as not "real police work" has been an interesting consequence of the government's review' (ibid. 2).

It is to be hoped that the worst excesses of the 'business' approach to policing have been left behind, with the government climb-down over the Sheehy report.[1] A return to old style policing is not an option and it seems likely that the era of financial constraints and increased accountability is here to stay. To some extent, the trend towards greater centralization is irreversible, as evidenced by the commissioning of the police national computer, the appointment of a national co-ordinator for the regional crime squads and the government's objective of increasing its influence on policing and security matters at the European level. It is neither possible nor desirable to resist these trends in an attempt to put the clock back, but it is important that the new structures for scrutinizing police activity are used to good effect.

A welcome sign that the policing of domestic violence is at last receiving serious appraisal, at least in Scotland, is indicated by the publication of a report by Her Majesty's Inspectorate of Constabulary for Scotland (1997) on this issue. The report provides an excellent case study both of the benefits of centralization and the spuriousness of creating artificial distinctions between core and peripheral policing functions, at a time when public perceptions of crime are changing rapidly. The authors point to the evidence that domestic violence has the highest rates of repeat victimization of any crime. In the United States 90 per cent of women killed by their partners were actively seeking outside help or attempting to leave.

On the issue of centralization, the report outlines a number of ways in which the sharing of information systems across police forces can be harnessed to improve both service delivery and crime detection. Based on a thematic inspection of all eight police forces in Scotland, the report draws on best practices found within particular forces to make a number of recommendations which include the following: that all forces nominate a senior officer to take responsibility for monitoring statistics on domestic violence, liaising with other organizations and informing policy at a strategic level; the use of repeat victimization statistics as a measure of the effectiveness of intervention; the issuing of mobile telephones or personal alarms to give a direct link to the police; the development of information systems to ensure that all relevant information about suspects is available to officers attending a domestic incident; and finally, the need to develop awareness of police responsibilities in relation to other vulnerable members of the household.

On the downside, the potentially harmful implications of centralization combined with a market ethos are raised in Liz Kelly *et al.*'s (1998) report on domestic violence for the Home Office Programme Development Unit, in which they refer to recent national changes in policing and criminal justice practices, particularly sectorization, charging standards and case disposal. They believe that these changes are potentially in tension with Home Office circular 60/1990 and local domestic violence policies, and they quote from an interview with a police officer who explains why the changes make the arrest of perpetrators of violence less likely:

> They say case disposal shouldn't have an influence on the decision you make at the scene – it shouldn't, but of course it does!...The goal is to ease the load on the CPS, decrease the number of cases going to court. It's not about equity in prosecuting cases, it's money saving, cost cutting, nothing else.
>
> (Interview with police officer, quoted in Kelly *et al.* 1998)

### Challenging cop culture

It is the entrenched nature of 'cop' culture (see Chapter 2) which appears to be at the root of police officer's resistance to any reform initiatives which involve changing long-established practices and attitudes (see for example McConville *et al.* 1991). Research shows that male officers are more likely to express traditional views of women's roles in society, for example that women's main duties should be confined to the domestic sphere and that women are unsuited to police work (Brown and Campbell 1991). Yet occupational culture is not monolithic and, as we have seen, there are individuals and groups within the police force who are increasingly prepared to challenge its dominant form (see also Fielding 1994). The particular style of policing associated with cop culture is increasingly less appropriate to meet the requirements of a modern police force. The bonds of solidarity forged between male officers who are securely within the culture may be functional for the survival of that group, but such exclusionary practices are damaging to the effective operation of the service as a whole.

The thematic inspection report *Developing Diversity in the Police Service* (HMIC 1995) recognizes the need to move towards a different style of policing. It emphasizes the importance of equal opportunities training as a tool for cultural change, which needs to 'run like a "golden thread" through all training programmes' (ibid. 45). However, a lack of commitment on the part of senior officers can lead to cynicism in the junior ranks. As one PC expressed it: 'We've only had equal opportunities training so that the chief can make us all legally liable and keep his name clear' (ibid. 45). It is clear from the report that such training should apply to all ranks and all areas of work and that it needs to be monitored and evaluated on a regular basis.

Chan's (1996) research into police culture in New South Wales showed that changes in recruitment and training were only partially successful in challenging the cultural 'tool-kit' which police officers utilized to make sense of their everyday experiences, as there was a lack of reinforcement once officers came into contact with 'real' police work. Her research also showed that when it came to the issue of police corruption, the determined efforts of the new Police Commissioner to stamp this out, backed by widespread community and political concern, were much more effective than similar initiatives against police racism and police abuse of power, which were not so strongly supported or enforced. This demonstrates the importance of the social, economic, legal and political sites in which policing takes place (Chan 1996). Changing police culture to bring it into line with the requirements of modern day policing is not impossible, but it does require a determined commitment on the part of government to eliminate discrimination by all possible means, both within the police service and in the wider society.

### Employment practices in the police

A central thesis of this book is that genuine and long-lasting improvements in service delivery will not be possible until the police put their own house in order. Until the composition of the force more closely resembles the general population in terms of gender, race and sexuality, stereotypical views held by police officers about women and minority groups are likely to persist. As Sandra Walklate (1996) points out, it is clear from existing research that 'people from ethnic minorities are simultaneously over-policed by their local police force and under-serviced by them when they find themselves to be the victims of crime' (ibid. 200). Similarly, sensitive policing of the gay and lesbian community is made much more difficult if homophobic attitudes are allowed to reign within the force unchecked. At the present time, gay and lesbian officers mostly keep their sexual identity hidden and there is no open debate on this issue (Kinsley Lord 1994).

There is a clear link between the requirement that sexual attacks are treated as serious crimes and the requirement that policewomen are treated as equal within the force. Equality means access to the same opportunities for recruitment, training and promotion and freedom from harassment. It means adopting employment practices sympathetic to the requirements of family life, for both men and women, and changing the perception of what constitutes 'real police work' so as to enhance the status of community policing and the protection of the vulnerable from violence, intimidation and abuse. The alternative, as Sandra Walklate (1996) argues, is to reconstitute Police Women's Departments in all but name, leaving the rest of police work untouched in both style and service delivery. For her, this is not a viable option and the findings presented in this book endorse this view.

The only alternative is for police forces to set themselves clear targets for the recruitment of women and ethnic minority officers to promote genuine 'diversity'. Once recruited, it will be vital to ensure that such officers are not isolated, but encouraged to apply for training courses and promotion and to move into the full range of specialist areas within the force. The introduction of family friendly employment practices and firm and fair anti-harassment policies would reduce wastage. The Equal Opportunities Commission has provided a useful summary of the benefits of equality and the costs of inequality, which should be imprinted on the brain of every police officer. The benefits include public confidence in a representative workforce, reduced staff turnover, improved morale and better service delivery. The costs include high staff turnover, low productivity, poor public image, wasted management time on grievances and the rising costs of litigation (EOC undated).

In the light of the harassment cases outlined in Chapter 2, it is clear that failure to take swift action on this issue can only mean that police forces throughout Britain face a nightmare scenario, in which the steady stream of tribunal cases alleging harassment becomes a torrent, as the tolerance levels of officers subjected to such treatment declines and the financial cost of settlements or awards escalates. The tragedy of allowing such a scenario to develop is that complainants would much prefer a satisfactory resolution of the problem, enabling them to continue their careers within the force, rather than being compelled to seek redress through litigation. As Tina Martin expresses it, 'they just want fairness, not hefty payouts' (interview with one of the authors, January 1998).

## From policing to criminal justice

Changing the priorities and practices of the police is the first step to reforming the criminal justice system if sexual violence against women and men is to be taken seriously. As we have argued elsewhere, if attempts on the part of the police to improve service delivery to complainants reporting rape and sexual assault are not reflected in far-reaching reforms at subsequent stages in the judicial process, then the fragile gains that have been made will be limited in their impact (Gregory and Lees 1994).

Joanna Shapland (1994) points out that the various agencies which make up the criminal justice system – and here she includes not only the police, prosecution, judiciary, court administration, probation and prisons, but also the Home Office, the Lord Chancellor's office and the Attorney General's Department – far from being parts of an interconnected system, act as independent 'fiefs' on a feudal model.

> Each fief retains power over its own jurisdiction and is jealous of its own workload and of its independence. It will not easily tolerate (or in some cases even permit) comments from other agencies about the way it conducts its business. This tendency is exacerbated and continued by the separate education and training of the professional workers for each fief, by their separate housing and by the hierarchical structure of promotion within fiefs, with little or no transfer between them.
>
> (Shapland 1994: 392)

This is a recipe for incoherence, inconsistency, secrecy and a defensive response to any questions from outsiders. Shapland's central concern is with victims caught up in this complex feudal web, with no one organization taking responsibility for ensuring that their needs are met.

Commenting on the improved services offered to complainants in sexual assault cases by the police and their total failure to impart this enthusiasm to other 'fiefs', she recommends a 'Round Table' of fiefs committed to the pursuit of justice.

The CPS is one of the most recently constructed 'fiefs', with its own workers, premises and philosophy. According to Williamson (1996), it is often perceived as an 'honest broker' in the middle of the adversarial process, a perception endorsed by the Royal Commission on Criminal Justice (1993), which favoured 'a system in which the roles of police, prosecutors and judges are as far as possible kept separate' (paragraph 1.14). Williamson takes issue with the Royal Commission and, like Shapland, argues for greater co-operation between the different parts of the system, believing that a more open system, while requiring 'higher levels of professionalism from all the disciplines involved' would 'make truth and justice more likely as outcomes than the present competitive system is capable of delivering' (Williamson 1996: 37).

Williamson goes further. He believes that the police, rather than the CPS, should hold the middle ground 'whilst the CPS and the defence slog it out in adversarial combat' (ibid. 37). The police should concentrate on their role as 'gatherers of fact and collectors of evidence' (ibid. 30). For Williamson, this is an essential part of the drive towards stamping out police corruption while enhancing the police role as peacekeepers and thereby shifting the focus of the front line agents of the criminal justice system from retributive to restorative justice.

## The feminization of social control

At one level, Williamson's analysis fits well with what Tamar Pitch (1985) calls 'the feminization of social control'. According to Heidensohn (1992), this means that certain organizations in post-war western societies have begun to adopt a less confrontational and more negotiated style of operation. As we argued in Chapter 2, if this is a 'feminine' approach to social control, one might expect more women to be employed as criminal justice professionals. In practice, we are confronted with the paradox that women are still very much in the minority throughout the criminal justice system. We saw that a mere 14 per cent of police officers are women, mostly concentrated in the lowest rank, and the legal profession presents an equally dismal picture, especially at the top end of the profession. A total of 71 per cent of solicitors on the Law Society's roll are male as are 78 per cent of barristers and 94 per cent of Queen's Counsels (QCs). Turning to the judges, the absence of women is even more marked. Taking the profession as whole, the judiciary is 90 per cent male and those women who are employed as judges are working mainly as assistant recorders, district judges, deputy district judges or stipendiary magistrates; even in these categories they are overwhelmingly outnumbered by men. At the top of the profession, the House of Lords judges and the Heads of Divisions are all men. There is one woman Appeal Court judge (out of 35) and seven High Court judges (out of 96) (EOC 1997).

The current system of appointments to the judiciary is as far removed from equal opportunities principles as it is possible to be, shrouded in secrecy, restrictive practices and a total lack of accountability. The Labour Party pre-election document referred to judicial appointments being made by 'a system of secretive patronage' which involves taking soundings from other judges and lawyers (Travis 1998). This system enables judges to clone themselves over and over again in making new appointments, reducing diversity to an absolute minimum, while maximizing conformity to conventional attitudes and traditional practices. It means that, for example, 'Not many human rights lawyers appear on the secret list which circulates among the judicial fraternity for their comment' (Kennedy 1992: 268).

Such secrecy has enabled such organizations as the freemasons to flourish unchallenged throughout the criminal justice system. Membership of the freemasons came to light during the investigation of the West Midland Serious Crime Squad who were involved in a number of miscarriages of justice. Criticism of the secret membership of such organizations by not only the police, but also by members of the judiciary, has led the Home Secretary to demand that the names of members working in the criminal justice system should be made public. This is in spite of reluctance on the part of the Lord Chancellor, Lord Irvine, who has fought to protect senior judges from this exposure (*Guardian*, 18 February 1998).

Before the election the Labour Party proposed the setting up of a judicial appointments commission which aimed to take the process of appointments out of the hands of the Lord Chancellor. The Labour Party Policy Handbook for candidates states:

> Labour will replace the current system of secretive patronage with a judicial appointments and training commission, independent of the Lord Chancellor's Department, to advise on all aspects of judicial appointments and training. It will oversee the advertise-ments of all judicial posts and selection procedures, will be

responsible for judicial performance appraisal and will ensure that complaints about judges' behaviour are taken seriously.

(see Travis 1998).

Although the Lord Chancellor conducted research into the American and Canadian models, which suggested that commissions were seen as a fairer way of appointing judges, such a commission has been rejected in Britain on the grounds that it would introduce the 'horrific' prospect of a repeat of the political battles by US senators over who should be confirmed as members of the Supreme Court. It is possible that the incorporation of the European Convention on Human Rights into British law will give judges a wider political role and that a different system of appointments which is more politically balanced will be introduced. However, there is no sign that changes will be anything more than cosmetic (such as the introduction of advertising posts for judges in February 1998, but where applicants must have served as barristers for ten years or circuit judges for two and are still appointed by the Lord Chancellor).

This system of appointment explains why so few women judges have been appointed. The majority of barristers are in any event conformist in training and outlook, but these practices ensure that anyone with more progressive inclinations, including the handful of women and members of ethnic minorities within the profession, will be discriminated against in the selection process. As Helena Kennedy argues, if women represented 30 per cent of the judiciary, tokenism would cease to function and a real difference would be felt. In order for such a radical transformation to be accomplished, far-reaching changes in the methods of recruitment and training for the profession would be needed and this in itself would ensure greater diversity within the judiciary and necessitate a cultural shift. Some of the more archaic practices associated with trials would be abandoned and the court would become a less intimidating place for witnesses. Sexual harassment by male judges and barristers of their colleagues is only beginning to come to light. In March 1998 the first judge was found guilty of sexual harassment of a pupil by a Bar disciplinary tribunal and resigned (Dyer 1998).

The concept of the feminization of social control as outlined in the work of Pitch (1985) and Heidensohn (1992) raises a second interesting paradox by suggesting that a more consensual, less adversarial approach to conflict resolution is in the ascendance in western societies. There can be no doubt that some victims of sexual violence would prefer a non-confrontational resolution of their situation, thereby avoiding the ordeal of a court appearance. There are some interesting parallels here with the sentiments expressed by women police officers involved in sexual harassment complaints; in both cases the chief concern is to secure a just outcome.

This raises the question of who is to mediate on behalf of the complainants and who is to monitor any settlement to ensure that agreements are honoured. In the case of bullying and harassment within the police force, as we have seen, a complete overhaul of the current grievance procedures is essential, shifting the emphasis from blaming the victim to resolving the dispute and exercising firm and fair discipline against the perpetrator. In the case of rape and sexual assault, a major overhaul of the existing arrangements for conducting rape trials is needed. Successful mediation can only work against the background of a much higher conviction rate. The present trend, in which the conviction rate has shrunk almost to vanishing point, means that the few defendants who are found guilty consider themselves to be extraordinarily unlucky and the vast majority who are acquitted consider their release justified. Unless the courts begin to reverse this trend and to send a clear message that male violence will not be condoned, complainants will continue to be denied justice, whether their cases are pursued through the courts or through the operation of a system of informal justice outside the formal court system.

If in the words of Williamson we leave the lawyers to 'slog it out in adversarial combat' (see above), while confining our reform initiatives exclusively to the police, progress will be severely limited. As our research evidence demonstrates, in the long run this is self-defeating, as it merely encourages more complainants to come forward and report sexual attacks, only for them to be denied justice at a later stage in the process. Nothing less than a radical overhaul of the entire criminal justice system is required, involving a transformation of the composition and culture of the various separate fiefdoms within it and an increased level of co-operation between them.

It is to be hoped that the recommendations of the Glidewell Report (1998) on the Crown Prosecution Service will go some way towards breaking down the separate fiefdoms within the criminal justice system. The report points to 'the failure of the police, the CPS and the courts to set overall objectives and agree the role and responsibility of each in achieving those objectives' (ibid. 6) and recommends the creation of 'one joint body at local level representing all the relevant criminal justice agencies' (ibid. 8; page numbers refer to the summary of the main report; see Review of the CPS 1998).

A major component of this cultural transformation has to be a marked shift of emphasis to the needs of complainants. In their evaluation report of the pilot project Domestic Violence Matters, Kelly *et al.* (1998) point to the failure of the criminal justice system as a whole to prioritize the safety of victims, particularly by not using remand in custody or pursuing breaches of bail vigorously enough. They refer to the approach adopted by the CPS, which does nothing to enable or encourage victim witnesses; starting from the presumption that women will withdraw, prosecutors act in such a way that in many cases this becomes a self-fulfilling prophesy. As an alternative approach, they point to the experience of other jurisdictions, which have seen the creation of trained prosecutors who specialize in domestic violence cases. They add that 'in some jurisdictions this has been extended to dedicated magistrates and judges and even the creation of domestic violence courts' (Kelly *et al.* 1998). They conclude:

> There has not been the movement in relation to law enforcement which the project initially hoped for. Whilst some responsibility for that must lie with the local criminal justice agencies, other factors were also at play. The attitudinal barriers and routine trivialising of domestic violence, which the police surveys documented, suffuses the police service, despite policy changes, and was echoed in some of the attitudes and practices of prosecutors, magistrates and judges.
>
> (Kelly *et al.* 1998)

## Rape law reform

### *Lessons from abroad*

There are difficulties with gaining rape convictions in all jurisdictions where sexuality is still defined by lawyers as appropriation and possession of the woman, where women's active sexuality is denied and where negotiated consent is not considered necessary (see Naffine 1994). This difficulty is reflected in the length of time it has taken to abolish the marital rape exemption, which in 1991 finally removed support for a husband's demand for the right to non-reciprocal sexual domination. When laws giving women substantial rights to the joint property on divorce had long come into force, the rape immunity law proved very difficult to abolish precisely because its abolition challenged the view of women as the possessions and passive objects of their husband's desires. Its abolition carries the clear implication that a woman does have a right to take an active rather than a passive sexual role and that acceptable forms of sexuality require the presence of mutual desire and consent, so absent from the definition of sexuality implied in rape trials.

There have, however, been significant and comprehensive reforms in other countries which are long overdue in Britain. In Michigan a package of reforms was introduced in the 1980s including the abolition of judicial discretion regarding sexual history evidence (except on two specified grounds), and the abolition of the need for corroboration or for proof of physical force. A major evaluation was conducted involving interviews with court officials, the police and rape crisis centre staff both before and after the new law was enacted. The effect was an increase in the rate of convictions as charged with a corresponding reduction in convictions for lesser offences. Also, trials became less of an ordeal for women as a consequence of these changes (see Adler 1987: 146).

In Canada too a package of reforms was introduced in the 1980s, including the controversial replacement of the crime of rape with three degrees of sexual assault. In 1983 an Act to Amend the Criminal Code (Sexual Assault) was passed which left the introduction of sexual history evidence to the discretion of judges. It required the defence to submit a written application containing details which would be heard in the absence of the jury and where witnesses could be called. Where such evidence was allowed, the judge would have to explain its relevance in writing (Temkin 1993: 18). According to Los (1990) feminists were not fully effective in lobbying for reform and those reforms that were introduced were in her view more a result of the introduction of the Charter of Rights and Freedoms rather than due to feminist pressure groups.

Legislation removing the discretion from judges regarding sexual character and sexual history evidence occurred fifteen years ago in Australia. The Crimes (Sexual Assault) Amendment Act and Cognate Act of 1981 in New South Wales, Australia, outlawed questioning about past sexual history which was seen as irrelevant to the woman's credibility, and all evidence produced as to the victim's sexual reputation of any kind was defined as 'inadmissible'. In the same way, complainants were prohibited from giving evidence of their own virginity at the time of the offence (Allen 1990). Additionally, the corroboration ruling was abolished. Judges are also required to warn against being prejudiced against women not reporting rape immediately. This has led to a greater willingness on the part of juries to convict and since these reforms, the level of arrests has increased and complaints are more actionable with different evidence and procedural provisions. It is, however, estimated that many cases still do not get to trial (Allen 1990: 230–1).

The system is, however, by no means perfect as is evident from a very thorough and critical research study *Heroines of Fortitude: The Experience of Women in Court as Victims of Sexual Assault* by Australia's Department of Women. This is the report of a 'Gender Bias and Law Project' (1996) which assesses the impact of reforms introduced by the Crimes Act 1990 in New South Wales. In spite of reformist legislation rendering, for example, evidence of sexual reputation completely inadmissible, the researchers found that evidence of the complainant's sexual reputation was still raised in 12 per cent of trials. Moreover in the 111 trials studied, sexual experience material was raised in 95 instances by the Crown and Defence. In some trials there were multiple instances of material concerning the prior sexual experience of the complainant ('Gender Bias and Law Project', Department of Women 1996: 10). The report also found that complainants were still discredited and attacked during cross-examination by questions and themes which were based on stereotyped views of appropriate behaviour of women complainants of sexual assault (1996: 7). In half the trials complainants were questioned about behaving in a sexually provocative way.

The most crucial reform recommended concerned the training provided by Law Schools and the Law Society, which the researchers argued should include information and research material on professional responsibility, clinical and skills training courses as well as substantive law courses. The report called for the Judicial Commission of New South Wales to provide education to judicial officers which included information and discussion about how to distinguish between sexual reputation and sexual experience, and how to apply tests of admissibility. We should take careful note of how vital it is that training, monitoring and accountability are written into any reforms if implementation of law reform is to be a reality. In the UK the appointment of special prosecutors, judges and police would also be required and the introduction of specialist training for all criminal justice professionals.

### Reforms in policing

Since the 1970s, feminist researchers and campaigners have challenged the division between the private and the public sphere and called on the police to adopt a law enforcement approach to domestic violence rather than refuse to take any action towards what were derisorily referred to as 'domestics' (see Stanko in Hanmer *et al.* 1989: 50). One of the first Canadian initiatives, referred to as the London Ontario model, was launched in 1982 and involved civil consultants backing up police policy. Jaffe *et al.* (1986) monitored the development of the new Ontario policy on the reporting of domestic violence by victims, neighbours and bystanders and reported that there was a 2,500 per cent increase in police use of assault charges in the handling of domestic violence calls. Although a policy directive from the Solicitor General encouraged a pro-arrest policy, as Kelly *et al.* (1998) point out, the current policy in Ontario is one of mandatory charge rather than mandatory arrest. These charges take the form of an 'appearance notice' (similar to a summons) which order the defendant to make a court appearance within a week or so. The charge is based not on the victim's wishes but on what happened. Trained prosecutors deal with such cases and a no-drop policy is enforced. The most important aspect was the back up of well resourced prevention and support services combined with monitoring and training. The Women's Directorate invested half a million dollars training 52 Crown Prosecutors. As we have seen, a pilot along these lines was introduced in Islington in 1991 but without the investment in the back up services which severely limited its effectiveness (Kelly *et al.* 1998).

In the United States Ferraro identifies three factors which combined during the 1980s to put pressure on police departments to treat domestic violence as a crime. These were the findings from social science research, pressure from the US Attorney General's Office and the National Institute of Justice, and the bringing of law suits against police departments for under-enforcement of the law. Sherman and Berk (1984) published their findings of a study of Minneapolis police in which they compared the policies of arrest, mediation and separation in domestic violence cases. They concluded that arrest was significantly more effective in deterring future violence than separation or mediation.

Nonetheless according to Ferraro (1993) wide variations in police practice still exist. Ferraro found a number of contradictions in the policy. Prejudiced views about women wasting police time and dropping charges prevailed. She found that every officer related cases where enormous resources had been invested before the complainant had then withdrawn. Where action had been taken against violent men, the same men were then granted custody and visiting rights to children. Ferraro concludes with these wise words:

> The data on implementing mandatory arrest suggest that it is difficult to change police responses to women battering and to eliminate discretion. Data on prosecution of assaults indicates that

most interpersonal violence, whether between strangers or intimates, is treated leniently by the courts. The obstacles to
increasing protection for women through the criminal justice
system are formidable and demand continuous monitoring and
involvement from feminists.

(Ferraro 1993: 175)

In New Zealand family courts have been set up and the Domestic
Violence Act 1995 has replaced non-molestation orders with the more
flexible and powerful protection orders. Penalties for breaching such
orders were increased to two years imprisonment. Additionally violent
parents are not entitled to custody or unsupervised access.
Rehabilitation programmes for children and survivors as well as perpetrators have been set up; for perpetrators they are compulsory (see
Ministry for Women's Affairs 1996). The most significant change is
that the police are more likely to make arrests than in the past.

### Reform at home

In England and Wales, there has been increasing publicity on the
falling conviction rate and the inadequacy of the judicial system to
protect women and children from violence. Recent television
programmes have highlighted a number of issues around which feminists have campaigned: rape in marriage (*World in Action* 1989),
lenient sentences in rape cases (BBC, *Panorama* July 1993) and the
scandal of serial rapists who escape justice only to rape many times
again (Channel 4, *Dispatches* 1994). The CPS has been criticized for
dropping too many cases, particularly when complainants then go on
to pursue a successful civil action (ITV, *The London Programme* 1993).
Judges have been criticized for lenient sentencing of men who kill their
wives (Channel 4, *Battered Britain* 1995) and Carlton *Thursday Night
Live* (October 1997) debated 'Is Sexual History Evidence Ever
Relevant?'. The attrition in domestic violence cases was also highlighted in two Channel 4 *Dispatches* documentaries, 'Men Behaving
Badly' (April 1998).

It is not only the media who have pointed to the ineffectiveness of
the judicial system. The police have in recent years become among the
most vociferous groups in favour of reform, as they are increasingly
frustrated by the failure of the system to convict suspects. In
September 1997 they took the unprecedented step of calling for
change at the Police Superintendents' Annual Conference in Bristol,
where the motion 'Are rape victims on trial?' was unanimously

supported. The conference called for urgent reform of the criminal justice system and supported limiting cross-examination of the complainant's sexual history.

In spite of this (in England and Wales) it appears that only small scale changes are on the agenda and then even their introduction is protracted. A good example is the proposed abolition of the right of defendants to cross-examine witnesses. The press gave widespread publicity to several recent cases where defendants have sacked their counsels and undertaken the cross-examination of their victims themselves. In the case of Julia Mason, her assailant Rallston Edwards cross-examined her for six days. He wore the same clothes as when he had repeatedly raped her (*Daily Telegraph*, 23 August 1996). Two months later, a Japanese woman who had been gang raped by five attackers was subjected to 12 days of cross-examination (*Guardian*, 7 September 1996). Shortly afterwards in November 1996, Michael Howard, then Conservative Home Secretary, announced that he intended to abolish the defendant's right to undertake his own defence in rape cases.

A year later, following the election of a Labour Government, still no change had been made in spite of two further cases where defendants had taken over their own defence. In the first case Floyd Bailey left his victim in tears after making her describe his genitals in graphic details. She later described her ordeal as 'being violated a second time' (Pallister 1998). After another case where the defendant, Milton Brown, who had been acquitted on four previous occasions, was allowed to cross-examine his victims for five days in the witness box, Jack Straw, the new Labour Home Secretary, promised a 'swift change in the law' to take forward the previous government's proposal (*Guardian*, 13 January 1998). Straw declared 'Women who have been raped should not be victims twice over. I set up an urgent review to identify ways to improve the treatment of vulnerable witnesses at every stage of the criminal justice process'. He said that he planned to put 'the interests of victims, not criminals, first' (see Lees 1997c).

A number of legislative reforms have been proposed, but at the time of writing in March 1998, nothing has actually been implemented. At this point it will be useful to outline exactly what has occurred in response to press, police and feminist concern about the failure of the judicial system to bring rapists to justice. At the instigation of Clare Short, then Shadow Minister for Women, a Labour Party Consultative document, *Peace at Home: Elimination of Domestic and Sexual Violence Against Women*, was published in October 1995 and launched at a day conference in February 1996 in London. It stated that Labour

Party policy was 'to take action to make the criminal justice system more responsive to the needs of women...to overhaul the current system of appointing and training judges, replacing decision making by the Lord Chancellor's office in secret with an independent judicial appointments commission which will take steps to ensure better representation for women' (ibid. 13). However, more than two years later, apart from a slightly more open system of appointing judges, very little appears to have changed.

On 12 June 1996, after questions had been asked in the House of Commons about why the conviction rate for rape had decreased so markedly (see Hansard Report: 355– 68),[2] three amendments to the Criminal Procedure and Investigation Bill were put forward by Jack Straw, the Shadow Home Secretary. The amendments concerned a prohibition on irrelevant questioning about the victim's past sexual history, the introduction of trial judges' warnings to ignore delays in reporting sexual offences and the strengthening of the 'similar fact' law whereby defendants could be charged with more than one offence at a time.

The most important amendment related to the admission of sexual history evidence. The new clause revised sections 1 and 2 of the Sexual Offences (Amendment) Act 1976 to provide important new protections from unjust, irrelevant and intrusive questioning of rape and sexual assault victims. Tessa Jowell, who had replaced Clare Short as Shadow Minister for Women, presented a spirited case for the amendments, arguing that:

> The proposals are based on the tried and tested formula of the 1981 New South Wales Act. The proposals set out in a new clause would establish for the first time clear and specific circumstances in which a judge may allow any questioning about the victim's sexual history. It requires the prosecution to seek permission to ask any suitable questions away from the jury, and requires the judge to state clearly in writing the questions that may be asked, and his reasons for giving such leave.
>
> (Hansard, 12 June: 365)

Although this tightened the procedure in so far as judges would be required to justify in writing the admission of sexual history and sexual character evidence, as we have seen, the evaluation of the Australian reforms shows that these have not been effectively implemented by judges in New South Wales (see 'Gender Bias and Law Project', Department of Women 1996). Given the record of British judges in ignoring earlier reforms on this issue (see Chapter 1), if such reforms were to be introduced here it would be essential to monitor them closely.

Mr Maclean MP, responding on behalf of the government, rejected the need for the amendments but did announce the setting up of a Home Office research project to investigate why the conviction rate had fallen so dramatically. This is unlikely to have much effect as previous Home Office studies (Smith 1989a, Grace, Lloyd and Smith 1992) have not led to any changes. Tessa Jowell was unimpressed:

> The length of the Minister's speech has served as an effective smokescreen for the fact that he has nothing to say. His lengthy diatribe about the defective nature of the new clauses is simply a way to side-step the real issues that they raise....The government's response to the new clause will be received by women across the country for what it represents: indifference, and a refusal to do anything about one of the most serious problems besetting women in the criminal justice system.
>
> (Hansard, 12 June: 365)

Following the election of a Labour government in May 1997, Prime Minister Tony Blair failed to set up a separate Ministry for Women and instead combined it with Social Security under the responsibility of Harriet Harman. However, there does appear to be commitment to reform the law on rape and in 1997 the Home Secretary, Jack Straw, set up a consultative body to draw up recommendations for law reform.

There is some cause for cautious optimism. As we have seen, a number of improvements have occurred in the past decade at both national and local level. Domestic violence units have been set up and the police have been directed to take domestic violence seriously. At local level more than 200 multi-agency forums have been established and Zero Tolerance campaigns have been launched in many Labour authorities. However, as Harwin (1997) documents, escaping from violence can be as hard as it was twenty years ago. Cuts in local authority spending are having a disastrous effect on rape crisis and counselling services and the Rape Crisis Federation, formed in 1996, is struggling to survive.

In response to the falling conviction rate, in 1997 a Campaign to End Rape was launched bringing together organizations such as Justice for Women, the Rape Crisis Federation (Wales and England), Action Against Child Sexual Abuse and a number of individuals. The aims of the campaign were to increase the conviction rate, ensure better treatment and representation of victims in court and change the law on consent. The campaign starts from the belief that consent must be negotiated, never presumed and points to Australia where, in the state of Victoria, it is the man who carries the burden of proving consent and evidence relating to the woman's sexual history is also outlawed

Overall, therefore, Britain lags behind other common law countries where far more sweeping, wide ranging reforms have been introduced. In June 1998, Jack Straw launched 'Speaking up for Justice', the report of the Interdepartmental Working Group on the treatment of vulnerable and intimidated witnesses in the criminal justice system (Home Office Interdepartmental Working Group 1998). Many of the recommendations have been included in the Crime and Disorder Act 1998, including the abolition of the defendant's right to take over his own defence in rape trials. It also introduces increased restrictions on the introduction of sexual history evidence, but without adequate training and monitoring, it is unlikely that such restrictions will be any more successful than the Sexual Offences (Amendment) Act 1976. Effective reform of the system depends crucially on the provision of adequate resources for training and retraining, on the provision of adequate support services and on ensuring that the perpetrators of violence are brought to justice and that women are protected from repeat victimization. This would also mean taking violence more seriously than property offences and theft, whereas at the present time the reverse is the case.

Several recent studies have pointed to the costs of domestic and sexual violence (see Stanko *et al.* 1997). The 1994 World Bank report *Violence Against Women: The Hidden Health Burden* found that in the US women who had been raped or beaten incur two and a half times the medical costs of women who have not been victimized (see *Peace at Home*, Labour Party 1995: 9). The costs of the effects of domestic violence on children are impossible to estimate but we know that witnessing violence can lead to a predisposition to violence and there is a growing body of evidence suggesting links between domestic violence and the physical and sexual abuse of children (Mullender and Morley 1994). Suzanne Snively (1995) estimated the cost of family violence in New Zealand to be at least $1.2 billion. The figure included the cost to individuals such as health care, loss of direct income, legal services and accommodation. It also included the government's costs through various portfolios including health, social welfare, justice and policing. If potential lost income and productivity are taken into account the real cost may be as high as $5.3 billion.

The basic underlying premise of the British adversarial system is to protect the rights of the defendant. In rape and sexual assault cases, the protection of defendants from false allegations predominates over the rights of complainants to obtain justice. Likewise, in cases of domestic violence, the rights of men as husbands and fathers is prioritized over the rights of women and children to be protected from violence. Conflict of interest is at the core of such court cases and the processes within the various judicial bodies, from the police through to the CPS, the judges and the Court of Appeal are weighted in favour of men. Unless legislative reforms are accompanied by an effective monitoring process, intensive training and procedures that render criminal justice institutions accountable, the likelihood of correcting this imbalance of power remains remote.

### Women's rights as human rights

There can be no doubt that the discourse of equal rights has in the past proved invaluable to the women's movement in campaigning for women's access to the same rights as men. While acknowledging that historically and politically such a strategy has proved significant, Carol Smart suggests that the rhetoric of rights is now exhausted and may even be detrimental, particularly where the demand is for a 'special' right for which there is no male equivalent (Smart 1989: 139). As she perceptively indicates, 'the resort to rights can be effectively countered by the resort to competing rights' (ibid. 145) and this is certainly the case in rape trials, where the rights of the complainant are counterposed to those of the defendant. As Longstaff and Neale (1997: 43) argue, 'the problem is not that defendants have too many rights but that victims have too few'.

We have suggested that it is possible to shift the balance so as to ensure that the complainant's version of events can be given due consideration, rather than distorted and discredited at every stage of the process and that this can be done without compromising the rights of the defendant. At the same time, we need to recognize the limitations of rights discourse, particularly its inability when considered in isolation to address inequalities of power between individuals and groups. The rhetoric of equal rights delivers formal equality, not substantive equality; treating people the same has different consequences for the parties involved and not everyone has the same possibility of ensuring access to his or her theoretical rights in practice.

In an international context, human rights discourse still has considerable leverage, because the oppression of women is so blatant the world over. In Britain, its leverage has declined as women have moved into the public sphere in ever-increasing numbers, giving rise to the belief that they have achieved equality and no longer require the special protection of the law. This book draws attention to the failure of the criminal justice system to protect the safety and dignity of the most vulnerable groups in the community. Against this background, we argue for a new concept of human rights which takes as its starting point the substantive inequalities between different individuals and groups and addresses the continuing widespread abuse of male power and control over the lives of women and children.

# Appendix

Information required from records of sexual assault on females: Holloway, Islington and Kings Cross Police Stations (September 1988 – September 1990)
N. of each record
Date

## 1. DETAILS OF SEXUAL OFFENCE

OFFENCE
        Rape
        Attempted Rape
        Indecent Assault
        Buggery
        Abduction
LOCATION
        Private place
        Victim's home
        Suspect's home
        Friend's home
        Party
        Other
        Public place
        Street
        Car park
        Vehicle: car, train, taxi
        Public house
        Wasteground
        Lift
        Other

TYPE OF SEXUAL ACTS
        Vaginal penetration
        Oral sex
        Digital penetration
        Penetration of inanimate object
        Buggery

DEGREES OF PHYSICAL VIOLENCE
ABH
GBH
Threatened
None

TYPE OF WEAPON
Please specify what type of weapon and if used or threatened

STATE OF VICTIM
Bruises
Cuts/scratches/minor abrasions

TIME LAPSE IN REPORTING FROM TIME OF RAPE
0–8 hours
9–24 hours
1–7 days
1–4 weeks
1–6 months
Over 6 months
RELATIONSHIP OF VICTIM TO SUSPECT
None
Knew by sight
Acquaintance
Close

DETAILS OF RELATIONSHIP IF KNOWN
Friend
Husband/cohabitee
Boyfriend
Former boyfriend
Former husband/cohabitee
Neighbour
Work colleague
Family friend
Relative

ETHNICITY OF VICTIM
1  2  3  4  5  6  (police categories)

AREA OF RESIDENCE

## 2. DETAILS OF SUSPECT

|  | Known | Not known |
|---|---|---|
| AGE if known | Below 16 | |
| | 16–20 years | |
| | 21–24 years | |

25–29 years
30–39 years
40–60 years
Over 60

## ETHNICITY OF SUSPECT
1   2   3   4   5   6   (police categories)

## AREA OF RESIDENCE

## PREVIOUS CONVICTIONS*

## 3. DETAILS OF PROCEDURE

## WHERE VICTIM TREATED/DETAINED

## REFERRALS
Victim Support
Social Services
Probation
Hospital
Criminal compensation
Other

## CRIMED/NO CRIMED
Please specify reason if no crimed

## SENT TO CPS
Yes          No      If no
a) Case no crimed
b) Suspect not found
c) Other

## FURTHER INFORMATION

---

* The police were not able/willing to supply us with information on the previous convictions of suspects.

# Notes

## 1 Introduction

1 Across India, 11,259 dowry related murders were officially registered during the three years 1995 to 1997, while only a handful of killers were brought to justice.
2 The danger of supporting reconciliation without adequate safeguards was tragically illustrated by the death of Vandana Patel, aged only 19, stabbed by her husband in Stoke Newington police station in 1991. She had agreed to meet him for talks about her marriage and had gone to the station because there was a domestic violence unit which she thought would provide a protective atmosphere.
3 The aim of the Act was also to make divorce less expensive to the state by reducing the cost to the Legal Aid Board.
4 Inspector Blair initiated police re-education in Britain following a visit to the United States, where police training in relation to rape, including the debunking of false allegation myths, had been introduced with some success.

## 2 Police culture and its contradictions

1 With the benefit of hindsight, it can be seen that the police force were better off without an exemption, as the armed forces exemption was successfully challenged under European law by two women dismissed from the armed services when they became pregnant. The Ministry of Defence had no choice but to admit liability and consequently to pay considerable sums in out of court settlements to women whose careers had been cut short as a result of the discriminatory policies.
2 In August 1993 the European Court of Justice ruled that the fixed upper limit on tribunal awards was contrary to European law, as the remedy had to be adequate to compensate for the loss and damage sustained (*Marshall v. Southampton and South West Hampshire Area Health Authority* [no.2], Case 271/91 [1993] IRLR 445). Following the removal of the compensation ceiling, within a short period of time average awards in discrimination cases rose by 45 per cent (Equal Opportunities Review Sept/Oct 1994, 57: 11).
3 See *Stewart* v. *Cleveland Guest (Engineering) Ltd* (1994) IRLR 440 and the discussion of this case in Rubenstein 1994 and Gregory 1995. The notion

that pin-ups of naked women are gender neutral is totally bizarre and in clear violation of the European Code of Practice.

## 3  Understanding attrition

1  Liz Kelly *et al.* (1998) experienced similar delays during their research, part of which involved tracking a sample of cases through police files and CPS files. Even though the study was an evaluation for the Home Office Development Unit, the request for access was referred to regional and national levels resulting in considerable delay. As CPS files are only available for 12 months, this meant redoing the process of identifying a sample of cases from the beginning.

2  McConville *et al.* (1991) make use of Herbert Packer's ideal types here. For Packer (1968), the crime control model is based on the principle that the fight against crime takes priority over all other considerations; offenders must be apprehended and punished by any efficient means. Due process principles focus instead on the need to protect the innocent from wrongful arrest and conviction, so there is an emphasis on the importance of checks, safeguards and reviewing procedures.

## 4  The decriminalization of rape?

1  This figure includes rapes of males as well as rapes of females, making direct comparison with earlier figures difficult. Very few cases of male rape progressed as far as a court hearing in 1996, although it is unclear how many were recorded (see Chapter 5).

2  Not until 1991 did the House of Lords confirm the legal possibility of marital rape in England and Wales (*R* v. *R* (1991) 2 WLR 1065). Our data refer to a time period prior to this decision.

3  Jennifer Temkin provides a detailed critical analysis of this case and considers its wider implications (Temkin 1993).

4  Unlike self-classification categories, when it is essential to find a form of description acceptable to all members of minority racial and ethnic groups, the police classification is based on a set of visual characteristics which some members of minority groups might well find offensive. The six categories are: White, White European, Negroid Black, Asian, Chinese Oriental and Arabic.

## 5  Male rape: the crime that can now speak its name

1  This documentary won the Royal Television prize for the best documentary of 1994.

2  The defendant, Richards, was sentenced to life imprisonment for the attempted rape of a 17 year old.

3  The New South Wales Women's Health and Sexual Assault Training and Education Unit recently produced a booklet on male sexual assault – (see Gender Bias and Law Project 1996).

## 6 Complainants' views of the police

1 Police Review, 28 Nov. 1975, quoted in London Rape Crisis Centre (1984: 141).

## 7 Complainants' views: the aftermath of sexual assault

1 Conducted by the Crime Victims Research and Treatment Centre.
2 Eleven women were interviewed but in two cases their view of the medical was not mentioned and in one further case the rape had occurred a year previously.
3 Funded by Gulbenkian, Barrow Cadbury, and the Allen Lane Foundation.

## 8 Conclusion

1 The Sheehy Inquiry into Police Responsibilities and Rewards was established in 1992 and reported the following year. It recommended the abolition of three ranks to rectify a top-heavy management structure, lower and locally determined starting salaries and allowances, performance related pay and fixed term appointments for all ranks. Following a well-orchestrated campaign from within the force, the Home Secretary backed down on the most contentious issues. Some ranks were abolished but he conceded that fixed-term appointments were inappropriate for ranks below superintendent and the recommendations in relation to pay were considerably watered down (Sheehy Report 1993, Leisham *et al.* 1996).
2 After widespread publicity given to the publication of Sue Lees' *Carnal Knowledge: Rape on Trial* (1997a), based on the consultancy work she undertook for the *Dispatches* programme 'Getting Away with Rape' (1994).

# Bibliography

Addison, N. (1996) 'The Public Deserves More', *The Times*, 30 April.

Adler, Z. (1987) *Rape on Trial*, London: Routledge.

—— (1991) 'Picking up the Pieces: A Survey of Victims of Rape', *Police Review* 31 May, pp. 1114–15.

—— (1992) 'Male Victims of Sexual Assault – Legal Issues' in G. Mezey and M. King (eds) *Male Victims of Sexual Assault*, Oxford: Oxford University Press, pp. 116–31.

Allen, J. (1990) *Sex and Secrets: Crimes involving Australian women since 1880*, Oxford: Oxford University Press.

Amir, M. (1971) *Patterns of Forcible Rape*, Chicago, IL: University of Chicago Press.

Anderson, L. (1997) 'Contact Between Children and Violent Fathers – In Whose Best Interests?', *Rights Of Women Bulletin*, summer: 30–7.

Anderson, R., Brown, J. and Campbell, E.A. (1993) *Aspects of sex discrimination in police forces in England and Wales*, London: Home Office Police Research Group.

Ashworth, A. ( 1992) *Sentencing and Criminal Justice*, London: Weidenfeld & Nicolson.

Bates, S. (1996) 'Paedophile Case Points to Police', *The Times*, 26 August.

*Battered Britain* (1995) 'Till Death Us Do Part', Channel 4, 11 October.

Becker, H. (1967) 'Whose Side Are We On?', *Social Problems* 14: 239–47.

Benson, M. and Walker, E. (1988) 'Sentencing the White Collar Offender', *American Sociological Review* 53: 294–302.

Benyon, J. (1989) 'A School for Men: An Ethnographic Case Study of Routine Violence in Schooling', in L. Barton and S. Walker (eds) *Politics and the Processes of Schooling*, 191–217, Milton Keynes: Open University Press.

Black, R. (1992) *Orkney A Place of Safety?*, Canongate Press.

Blair, I. (1985) *Investigating Rape*, London: Croom Helm.

Block, B., Corbett, C. and Peay, J. (1993) *Ordered and Directed Acquittals in the Crown Court*, Royal Commission Research Study 15, London: HMSO.

Boggan, S. and Marks, K. (1998) 'In the Courts: Judge says sex killer Farrant should stay behind bars for life', *Independent*, January 30.

Bottomley, A. and Coleman, C. (1981) *Understanding Crime Rates*, London: Saxon House.

Bourlet, A. (1990) *Police Intervention in Marital Violence*, Milton Keynes: Open University Press.

Bourque, L. (1989) *Defining Rape*, Durham and London: Duke University Press.

Box-Grainger, J. (1986) 'Sentencing Rapists' in R. Matthews and J. Young, *Confronting Crime*, London: Sage, pp. 31–52.

Brewer, J.D. (1991) 'Hercules, Hippolyte and the Amazons – or policewomen in the RUC', *British Journal of Sociology* 42: 231–247.

*British Crime Survey* (1996) London: Home Office.

Brooks, L. (1998) 'The Ultimate Designer Date Rape Drug?', *Guardian*, 13 January.

Brown, B., Burman, M. and Jamieson, L. (1992) *Sexual History and Sexual Character Evidence in Scottish Sexual Offence Trials*, Edinburgh: Scottish Office Central Research Unit Papers.

Brown, J. (1998) 'Aspects of Discriminatory Treatment of Women Police Officers Serving in Forces in England and Wales', *British Journal of Criminology* 38 (2): 265–82.

Brown, J. and Campbell, E.A. (1991) 'Less than Equal', *Policing* 7 (4): 324–33.

Brown, J., Campbell, E.A. and Fife-Schaw, C. (1995) 'Adverse Impact Experienced By Police Officers Following Exposure to Sex Discrimination and Sexual Harassment', *Stress Medicine* 11: 221–8.

Brown, M. (1992) 'It Could Happen To Any Man, Any Time', *Observer*, 30 October.

Brownmiller, S. (1978) *Against Our Will*, Harmondsworth: Penguin.

Bryant, L., Dunkerley, D. and Kelland, G. (1985) 'One of the Boys?', *Policing* 1 (4): 236–44.

Burke, M.E. (1993) *Coming Out of the Blue*, London: Cassells.

Butler-Sloss, Lord Justice (1988) *Report of the Judicial Inquiry into Child Abuse in Cleveland 1987*, Cm 412, London: HMSO.

Campbell, B. (1988, 1997) *Unofficial Secrets: Child Sexual Abuse – The Cleveland Case*, London: Virago.

Campbell, D. (1997) 'Come in Bonky, Porky and Gonzo, your time is up', *Guardian*, 13 November.

Centre for Police Studies (1989) *The Effect of the Sex Discrimination Act on the Scottish Police Service*, Strathclyde: University of Strathclyde.

Chambers, G. and Millar, A. (1983) *Investigating Sexual Assault*, Edinburgh: Scottish Office Central Research Unit Study, HMSO.

—— (1986) *Prosecuting Sexual Assault*, Edinburgh: Scottish Office Central Research Unit Study, HMSO.

Chan, J. (1996) 'Changing Police Culture', *British Journal of Criminology* 36 (1): 109–34

Clark, A. (1987) *Men's Violence, Women's Silence*, London: Pandora.

Cohen, J. (1993) 'Seeing Red About the Boys in Blue', *Guardian*, 25 August.

Connell, R.W. (1987) *Gender and Power*, Cambridge: Polity.
—— (1995) *Masculinities*, Cambridge: Polity Press.
Corbett, C. (1987) 'Victim Support Services to Victims of Serious Sexual Assault', *Police Surgeon* 32: 6–16.
Coward, R. (1997) 'Sign of the Crimes', *Guardian*, 24 July.
Coxell, A. and King, M. (1996) 'Male Victims of Rape and Sexual Abuse', *Sexual and Marital Therapy* 11: 297–308.
Coxell, A., King, M., Mezey, G. and Gordon, D. (forthcoming) *Prevalence of Unwanted and Under-age Sexual Experiences in Adult Men: A National Study*.
Cretney, A. and Davis, G. (1996) 'Prosecuting Domestic Assault', *Criminal Law Review*, 162–74.
—— (1997) 'Prosecuting Domestic Assault: Victims Failing Courts, or Courts Failing Victims?', *The Howard Journal* 36 (2): 146–57.
Cromack, V. (1995) 'The Policing of Domestic Violence: An Empirical Study', *Policing and Society* 5: 185–99.
Crown Prosecution Service (1992) *Code for Crown Prosecutors*, London: CPS.
—— (1994a) *Code for Crown Prosecutors*, London: CPS.
—— (1994b) *Annual Report 1993–4*, London: HMSO.
—— (1995) *Discontinuance Survey*, London: CPS.
—— (1996) *An Extraordinary Memorandum for Use in Connection with the Code for Crown Prosecutors*, London: CPS.
Crown Prosecution Service Inspectorate (1998) *Report on Cases Involving Child Witnesses*, London: CPS Inspectorate.
Daly, K. and Stephens, D. (1995) 'The "Dark" Figure of Criminology' in N. H. Rafter and F. Heidensohn (eds) *International Perspectives in Criminology*, Buckingham: Open University Press, pp.189–215.
Daly, M. and Wilson, M. (1993) 'Spousal Homicide Risk and Estrangement', *Violence and Victims* 8: 13–60.
Davis, A. (1981) *Women, Race and Class*, New York: Random House.
Davis, N. (1985) 'The Re-Education of Police Personnel in the Investigation of Sexual Offences', *Police Surgeon* 28: 8–14.
*Dispatches* (1994) 'Getting Away with Rape', First Frame, Channel 4, 6 February.
—— (1995) 'Male Rape', Platinum Productions, Channel 4, 17 May.
—— (1998) 'Men Behaving Badly', First Frame, Channel 4, 16 and 23 April.
Dunhill, C. (ed.) (1989) *The Boys in Blue: Women's Challenges to the Police*, London: Virago.
Dyer, C. (1998) 'Judge found guilty of sexual harassment quits bench', *Guardian*, 3 March.
Edwards, S. (1989) *Policing 'Domestic' Violence: Women the Law and the State*, London: Sage.
Equal Opportunities Commission (1997) *Facts about Women and Men in Great Britain*, Manchester: EOC.

—— (undated) *The Business Case for Equal Opportunities in the Police Service*, Manchester: EOC.

Equal Opportunities Commission/Metropolitan Police (1989) *Managing to Make Progress*, London: Metropolitan Police.

European Commission (1992) 'Recommendation on the Protection of the Dignity of Women at Work and Code of Practice on Measures to Combat Sexual Harassment', *Official Journal of the European Communities* 35 (L.49), Luxembourg.

European Parliament (1986) Report on behalf of the Committee on Women's Rights on *Violence Against Women* (d'Ancona Report), A2-44/86, Luxembourg.

*Everyman* (1990) 'No Great Trauma', BBC2, 16 Sept.

Fagan, J. (1996) *The Criminalization of Domestic Violence: Promises and Limits*, Washington DC: National Institute of Justice.

Faizey, M. (1994)'Let down by the Law', *Guardian*, 20 August.

Faragher, T. (1985) 'The Police Response To Violence Against Women in the Home' in J. Pahl (ed.) *Private Violence and Public Policy*, Routledge & Kegan Paul, pp. 110–24.

Ferraro, K. (1989) 'The Legal Response To Woman Battering In The US' in J. Hanmer, J. Radford and E. Stanko (eds) *Women, Policing and Male Violence*, London: Routledge, pp. 155–84.

—— (1993) 'Cops, Courts and Woman Battering' in P. Bart and E. Moran (eds) *Violence Against Women*, London: Sage, pp. 165–77.

Fielding, N. (1994) 'Cop canteen culture' in T. Newburn and E.A. Stanko (eds) *Just Boys Doing Business? Men, Masculinities and Crime*, London: Routledge, pp. 46–63.

Fionda, J. (1995) 'The Scottish Procurator Fiscal Service: The Reluctant Sentencers' in *Public Prosecutors and Discretion: A Comparative Study*, Clarendon Press.

Foley, M. (1994) 'Professionalizing the Response to Rape' in C. Lupton and T. Gillespie (eds) *Working Out*, London: Macmillan, pp. 39–54.

—— (1996) 'Who is in Control?: Changing Responses to Women Who Have Been Raped And Sexually Abused' in M. Hester, L. Kelly and J. Radford (eds) *Women, Violence and Male Power*, London: Routledge, pp. 166–75.

Frohmann, L. (1991) 'Discrediting Victims: Allegations of Sexual Assault – Prosecutorial Accounts of Case Rejections', *Social Problems* 38 (2).

Gender Bias and Law Project (1996) *Heroines of Fortitude: The Experiences of Women in Court as Victims of Sexual Assault*, Department for Women, New South Wales, Australia.

Gillespie, T. (1996) 'Rape crisis centres and "male rape": a face of the backlash' in M. Hester, L. Kelly and J. Radford (eds) *Women, Violence and Male Power*, Milton Keynes: Open University Press, pp. 148–65.

Grace, S. (1995) *Policing Domestic Violence in the 1990s*, Home Office Research Study No. 139, London: HMSO.

Grace, S., Lloyd, C. and Smith, L. (1992) *Rape: From Recording to Conviction*, London: Home Office Research Unit.

Gregory, J. (1995) 'Sexual Harassment: Making the Best Use of European Law', *European Journal of Women's Studies* 2: 421–40.

Gregory, J. and Lees, S. (1994) 'In Search of Gender Justice : Sexual Assault and the Criminal Justice System', *Feminist Review* 48 (autumn): 80–93.

Groth, A.N. (1979) *Men Who Rape*, New York: Plenum.

Grubin, D. and Gunn, J. (1990) *Imprisoned Rapists and Rape*, London: Home Office Research Unit.

Hague, G. and Malos, E. (1993) *Domestic Violence: Action for Change*, Cheltenham: New Clarion Press.

Halford, A. (1993) *No Way up the Greasy Pole*, London: Constable.

Hall, R. (1985) *Ask Any Woman*, London: Falling Wall Press.

Hanmer, J. (1994) *Policy Developments and Implementation Seminars: Pattern of Agency Contact with Women*, Research Paper No. 12, Violence, Abuse and Gender Relations Research Unit, University of Bradford.

Hanmer, J. and Saunders, S. (1990) *Women, Violence and Crime Prevention: a study of changes in police policy and practices in West Yorkshire*, Violence, Abuse and Gender Relations Study Unit Research Paper 1, Bradford: Department of Social Studies Bradford University.

Hanmer, J., Radford, J. and Stanko, E. (eds) (1989) *Women, Policing and Male Violence*, London: Routledge.

Hansard (Parliamentary Debates) House of Commons, London: HMSO.

Harris, J. (1997) *The Processing of Rape Cases by the Criminal Justice System: Interim Report*, London: Home Office.

Harwin, N. (1997) *Vulnerable and Intimidated Witnesses: Improving Safety and Protection for Women and Children Experiencing Domestic Violence*, Bristol: Women's Aid Federation.

Hearn, J. *et al. Violence by Organisations, Violence in Organisations, and Organisational Responses to Violence*, University of Bradford Research Paper 2.

Heidensohn, F. (1992) *Women in Control: The Role of Women In Law Enforcement*, Oxford: Oxford University Press.

Heilbron Committee (1975) *Report on the Advisory Group on the Law on Rape*, Cmnd 6352, London: HMSO.

Her Majesty's Inspectorate of Constabulary (1992) *Equal Opportunities in the Police Service*, London: Home Office.

—— (1995) *Developing Diversity in the Police Service*, London: Home Office.

Her Majesty's Inspectorate of Constabulary for Scotland (1997) *Hitting Home: A Report on the Police Response to Domestic Violence*, Edinburgh: HMSO.

Hester, M. and Radford, L. (1996) 'Domestic Violence and Access Arrangements in Denmark and Britain', *Journal of Social Welfare and Family Law* 1: 57–70.

Hirsch, A. and Roberts, J. (1997) 'Racial Disparity in Sentencing: Reflections on the Hood Study', *Howard Journal* 36 (3): 227–36.

Holdaway, S. (1996) *The Racialization of British Policing*, Basingstoke: Macmillan.

Holmes, K. and Williams, J. (1979) 'Problems and Pitfalls of Rape Victims Research: An Analysis of Selected and Pragmatic Concerns', *Victimology* 4: 17–28.

Holmstrom, L. and Burgess, A. (1978) *The Victim of Rape: Institutional Reactions*, New York: John Wiley & Sons.

Home Affairs Select Committee on Domestic Violence (1993) *Domestic Violence*, Vols I and II, London: HMSO.

Home Office (1990) *Victim's Charter: A Statement of the Rights of Victims of Crime*, London: Home Office.

—— (1993a) 'The Long Term Needs of Victims: A Review of the Literature', *Research and Planning Unit Paper 80*.

—— (1993b) *White Paper on Police Reform*, Cm 2281, London: HMSO.

—— (1996) *The Victim's Charter: A Statement of the Service Standards for Victims of Crime*, London: Home Office.

Home Office Bulletin (1989) *Statistics on Offences of Rape 1977–1987*, Home Office 4/89.

Home Office Interdepartmental Working Group (1998) *Speaking up for Justice: The Report of the Interdepartmental Working Group on the Treatment of Vulnerable and Intimidated Witnesses in the Criminal Justice System*, London: Home Office.

Home Office Statistical Bulletin (1995).

Home Office Statistics (1993 and 1996) Available from Home Office Research and Statistics Department.

Hugill, B. (1996) 'Paedophilia is a Billion Dollar Business', *Observer*, 25 August.

Jaffe, P., Wolfe, P., Telford, A. and Austin, G. (1986) 'The impact of police charges in incidents of wife abuse', *Journal of Family Violence* 1: 37–49.

Jefferson, J.M. and Shapland, J. (1990) 'Criminal Justice and the Production of Order and Control: Trends since 1980 in the UK', Paper presented to *GERN Seminar* on the Production of Order and Control, Paris: CESDIP.

Johnson, L. (1998) 'Harrowing Court Ordeal of Battered Wives to End', *Observer*, 8 February.

Jones, S. (1986) *Policewomen and Equality*, Basingstoke: Macmillan.

Jones, T., Maclean, B. and Young, J. (1986) *The Islington Crime Survey*, London: Gower.

Joutsen, M. (1987) *The Role of the Victim of Crime in European Criminal Justice Systems*, Helsinki: HEUNI.

Kelly, L. (1988) *Surviving Sexual Violence*, Cambridge: Polity.

Kelly, L., Bindel, J., Burton, S., Butterworth, D., Cook, K. and Regan, L. (1998) *Domestic Violence Matters: A Developmental Study*, Home Office Research Study 188, London: The Stationery Office.

Kennedy, H. (1992) *Eve was Framed*, London: Chatto & Windus.

Kenway, J. (1995) 'Masculinities in Schools: Under siege, on the defensive and under control?', *Discourse* 16 (1) pp. 58–79.

King, J. and Brown, J. (1997) *Gender Differences in Police Officers' Attitudes Towards Rape: Implications for Investigative Practice*, Dept. of Psychology, University of Surrey.

King, M. (1992) *Male Rape in Institutional Settings*, Oxford: Oxford University Press.

Kinsey, A. (1948) *Sexual Behaviour in the Human Male*, Philadephia, PA: Saunders.

Kinsley, Lord (1994) *The Metropolitan Police Service: Development of an Equal Opportunities Strategy*, London: Kinsley Lord Consultants.

Koss, M. and Harvey, M. (1988) *The Rape Victim: Clinical and Community Interventions*, London: Sage.

Labour Party (1995) *Peace at Home: A Labour Party Consultation on the Elimination of Domestic and Sexual Violence Against Women*, London: National Office.

LaFree, G. (1980) 'The Effect of Sexual Stratification by Race on Official Reactions to Rape', *American Sociological Review*, 45 (5): 842–52.

—— (1982) 'Male Power and Female Victimization: Towards A Theory Of Interracial Crime', *American Journal of Sociology*, 88: 311–28.

—— (1989) *Rape and Criminal Justice*, Belmont, CA: Wadsworth.

Lea, J. (1992) 'The Analysis of Crime' in Young and Matthews (eds) *Rethinking Criminology: The Realist Debate*, Sage.

Lees, S. (1993) 'Judicial Rape', *Women's Studies International Forum* 16 (1): 11–36, Pergamon.

—— (1997a) *Carnal Knowledge: Rape on Trial*, Harmondsworth: Penguin.

—— (1997b) *Ruling Passions*, Buckingham: Open University Press.

—— (1997c) 'A Fair Deal', *Guardian*, 11 November.

Lees, S. and Gregory, J. (1993) *Rape and Sexual Assault: A Study of Attrition*, London: Islington Council.

Leidholdt, D. (1996) 'Sexual Trafficking of Women in Europe' in *Sexual Politics in the European Union: the New Feminist Challenge*, Berghahn Books, pp. 83–95.

Leishman, F., Loveday, B. and Savage, S.P. (1996) *Core Issues in Policing*, London: Longman.

Lewington, F. (1991) 'Police Surgeons and Rape Victims', *British Medical Journal* 303: 713.

Lloyd, C. and Walmsley, R. (1989) *Changes in Rape Offences and Sentencing*, Home Office Research Study No. 105, London: HMSO.

*London Programme* (1993) 'The Crown Prosecution Service', Thames TV, 13 August.

London Rape Crisis Centre (1984) *Sexual Violence: The Reality for Women*, London: The Women's Press.

Longstaff, L. and Neale, A. (1997) 'The Convicted Rapist Feels Unlucky – Rarely Guilty', *The Times*, 18 November.

Los, M. (1990) 'Feminism and rape law reform' in L. Gelsthorpe and A. Morris, *Feminist Perspectives in Criminology*, Milton Keynes: Open University Press, pp. 160–72.

Maddock, O. and Scott, H. (1995) *Reach: Evaluation Report*, Newcastle: University of Northumbria.

Maguire, M. and Corbett, C. (1987) *The Effects of Crime and the Work of Victim Support Schemes*, Aldershot: Gower.

Mama, A. (1989) *The Hidden Struggle*, London Race and Housing Research Unit and Runneymede Trust; repr. 1996 London: Whiting & Birch.

Martin, C. (1996) 'The Impact of Equal Opportunities Policies on the Day-to-day Experiences of Women Police Constables', *British Journal of Criminology* 36 (4): 510–28.

Martin, T.M. (1996) *Rocking the Boat*, unpublished MA Dissertation, University of Leicester.

Mawby, R.I. and Walklate, S. (1994) *Critical Victimology*, London: Sage.

Mayhew, P (1984) 'The British Crime Survey 1st Report', Home Office Research and Planning Unit, No. 85, HMSO.

McBarnet, D. (1981) *Conviction*, London: Macmillan.

McCarthy, M. (1996) 'Sexual experiences and sexual abuse of women with learning disabilities' in M. Hester, L. Kelly and J. Radford (eds) *Women, Violence and Male Power*, Milton Keynes: Open University Press, pp. 119–29.

McColgan, A. (1996) 'Common Law and the Relevance of Sexual History Evidence', *Oxford Journal of Legal Studies* 16: 275–307.

—— (1997) *The Case for Taking the Date Out of Rape*, London: Harper Collins.

McConville, M., Sanders, A. and Leng, R. (1991) *The Case For The Prosecution: Police Suspects And The Construction Of Criminality*, London: Routledge.

McMullen, R.J. (1990) *Male Rape: Breaking the Silence on the Last Taboo*, London: Gay Men's Press Publishers.

Metropolitan Police (1986a) *Working Party on Domestic Violence Report*, London: Metropolitan Police.

—— (1986b) *Equal Opportunities Guidelines for Police Managers*, London: Metropolitan Police.

—— (1995) *The Investigation of Serious Sexual Assaults: Police guidelines for Investigators and Chaperones*, London: New Scotland Yard.

Mezey, G. and King, M.B. (eds) (1992) *Male Victims of Sexual Assault*, Oxford: Oxford University Press.

Mezey, G. and Taylor, P. (1988) 'Psychological Reaction of Women who have been Raped: A Descriptive and Comparative Study', *British Journal of Psychiatry* 152: 330–9.

Ministry for Women's Affairs (1996), Press release on changes to the Domestic Violence Act 1996, Wellington: New Zealand.

Moody, S and Tombs, J. (1983) 'Plea Negotiations in Scotland', *Criminal Law Review*, pp. 297–307.

Mooney, J. (1993) *Hidden Figure: Domestic Violence in North London*, London: Islington Council.

Moran, R.A. (1994) 'Personal Responsibility Without Personal Control', Paper given at the *British Sociological Association Annual Conference*, Preston.

Morley, R. and Mullender, A. (1994) *Preventing Domestic Violence to Women*, Home Office Research Group, Crime Prevention Unit Series, Paper 48.

Moxon, D. 1988 *Sentencing Practice in the Crown Court*, Home Office Research Study No. 103, HMSO.

Mullender, A. (1996) *Rethinking Domestic Violence*, Routledge.

Mullender, A. and Morley, R. (1994) *Children Living with Domestic Violence: Putting Men's Abuse of Women on the Child Care Agenda*, London: Whiting & Birch.

Myers, P. (1997)'An Unfair Cop', *Guardian*, G2 supplement, 23 September, p. 17.

Naffine, N. (1994) 'Possession: Erotic Love and the Law on Rape', *Modern Law Review*, 57 (1): 10–37.

National Children's Home (1997) *The Age of Anxiety*, London: Action for Children.

National Society for the Prevention of Cruelty to Children (1992) *Child Abuse Trends*, London: NSPCC.

National Women's Council of Ireland (1996) *Victims of Sexual and Other Crimes of Violence Against Women and Children*, Dublin Report of the Working Party on the Legal and Judicial Process.

National Women's Study (1992) *Rape in America: A Report to the Nation*, Crime Victims Research and Treatment Centre.

Newburn, T. (1993) 'The Long-term Needs of Victims', *Research and Planning Unit Paper 80*, London: Home Office.

Nielsen, T. (1983) 'Sexual Assault of Boys: Current Perspectives', *Personnel and Guidance Journal*, 62: 139–42.

O'Hara, M.(1997) 'Prostitution: Developing Feminist Law Reform', *Rights of Women Bulletin*, summer: 11–21.

Oxford University Students Union (1994) *Sexual Harassment Survey*.

Paddison, L. (1992) 'Halford: Tip of an Iceberg?', *Personnel Management*, September.

Pallister, D. (1998) 'Rapist Who Tortured Girlfriend Sentenced to Five More Years', *Guardian*, 17 January.

*Panorama* (1993) 'The Rape of Justice', BBC1, 16 July.

Pickard, J. (1995)'Pulling Rank on the Boys in Blue', *People Management*, 24 August: pp. 24–5.

Pitch, T. (1985) 'The Feminization of Social Control' *Research in Law, Deviance and Social Control* 7, autumn.

Polk, K. (1985) 'A Comparative Analysis of Attrition of Rape Cases', *British Journal of Criminology* 25 (2) July: 280–4.

Poole, E.D. and Pogrebin, M.R. (1988) 'Factors Affecting The Decision to Remain in The Police: A Study of Women Officers', *Journal of Police Science Administration* 16: 46–55.

*Public Eye* (1992) 'Hidden from View, Hidden from Justice', BBC2, February.

Radford, J. (1987) 'Policing Male Violence – Policing Women' in J. Hanmer and M. Maynard (eds) *Women, Violence and Social Control*, Basingstoke: Macmillan, pp. 30–45.

—— (1989) 'When Legal Statements Become Pornography: A New Cause For Concern in the Treatment of Rape in the Legal Process', *Rights of Women Bulletin*, autumn: 5–7.

—— (1996) 'Breaking Up is Hard To Do', *Trouble and Strife* 34 (Winter): 12–20.

Radford, J. and Stanko, E. (1996) 'Violence Against Women and Children: The Contradictions of Crime Control under Patriarchy' in M. Hester, L. Kelly and J. Radford (eds) *Women, Violence and Male Power*, Milton Keynes: Open University Press, pp. 657–80.

Radio 4, *World Tonight Special* (1996) 'Can't You Take a Joke?', 26 September.

Reiner, R. (1978) *The Blue Coated Worker*, Cambridge: Cambridge University Press.

—— (1992) *The Politics of the Police*, Brighton: Wheatsheaf.

The Review of the Crown Prosecution Service (The Glidewell Report) (1998) Cm 3960, London: The Stationery Office.

The Review of the Crown Prosecution Service: Summary of The Main Report with Conclusions and Recommendations (1998) Cm 3972, London: The Stationery Office.

Rights of Women (1994) *Rights of Women Bulletin*, spring.

—— (1997) 'Best Interests Campaign', London.

Robbins, D. (1986) *Wanted: Railman*, Equal Opportunities Commission Research Series, London: HMSO.

Roberts, C. (1989) *Women and Rape*, Brighton: Harvester Wheatsheaf.

Robertshaw, P. (1994) 'Sentencing Rapists: First Tier Courts in 1991–92', *Criminal Law Review*, 1994: 343–5.

Rodkin, L., Hunt, E. and Cowan, S. (1982) 'A Man's Support Group for Significant Others of Rape Victims', *Journal of Marital & Family Therapy* 8: 91–7.

Rose, D. (1996a) *In the Name of the Law: The Collapse of Criminal Justice*, London: Jonathan Cape.

—— (1996b) 'When Justice Takes a Walk', *Guardian*, 19 November.

Rozenberg, J. (1987) *The Case for the Crown: the Inside Story of the Director of Public Prosecutions*, Wellingborough: Thorsons Public Co.

Rubenstein, M. (1994) 'Pin-ups and Sexual Harassment', *Equal Opportunities Review* 57: 38–42.

Rumney, P. (1999) 'When Rape isn't Rape', *Oxford Journal of Legal Studies* 19 (2).

Rumney, P. and Morgan-Taylor, M. (1997) 'Recognizing the Male Victim: Gender Neutrality and the Law on Rape Pt1 & Pt2', *Anglo-American Law Review* 26: 198–356.

Rush, F. (1990) 'The Many Faces of the Backlash' in D. Leidholdt and J.G. Raymond (eds) *The Sexual Liberals and the Attack on Feminism*, Oxford: Pergamon Press.

Sanders, A. (1994) 'Constructing the Case for the Prosecution' in N. Lacey (ed.) *A Reader in Criminal Justice*, Oxford Readings in Socio-legal Studies, Oxford University Press.

Saward, J. (1990) *Rape: My Story*, London: Bloomsbury.

Scott, S. and Dickens, A. (1989) 'Police and the Professionalization of Rape' in C. Dunhill (ed.) *The Boys in Blue*, London: Virago, pp. 80–91.

Scully, D. (1990) *Understanding Male Violence*, London: Unwin.

Seabrook, M. (1990) 'Power Lust', *New Statesman & Society*, 27 April 1990.

Shapland, J. (1994) 'Fiefs and Peasants: Accomplishing Change for Victims in the Criminal Justice System' in N. Lacey (ed.) *A Reader in Criminal Justice*, Oxford Readings in Socio-legal Studies, Oxford University Press.

Sheehy Report (1993) *Inquiry into Police Responsibilities and Rewards*, London: HMSO.

Sherman, L.W. and Berk, R.A. (1984) 'The Specific Deterrent Effects of Arrest for Domestic Assault', *American Sociological Review* 49: 261–72.

Sim, J., Scraton, P. and Gordon, P. (1987) 'Introduction' in P. Scraton (ed.) *Law, Order and the Authoritarian State*, London: Routledge.

Skidmore, P. (1995) 'Telling Tales: Media Power, Ideology and the Reporting of Child Sexual Abuse in Britain' in D. Kidd-Hewitt and R. Osborne (eds) *Crime and the Media*, London: Pluto Press.

Smart, C. (1989) *Feminism and the Power of Law*, London: Routledge.

Smith, D.J. and Gray, J. (1985) *Police and People in London: the PSI Report*, Aldershot: Gower.

Smith, G. (1980) 'Rape' (paper presented to the Association of Police Surgeons' Symposium), *Police Surgeon* 17: 46–56, quoted in Temkin (1996).

Smith, L. (1989a) *Concerns about Rape*, Home Office Research Study No. 106, HMSO.

—— (1989b) *Domestic Violence: An Overview*, London: HMSO.

Snively, S. (1995) *The New Zealand Economic Cost of Family Violence*, Wellington: Coopers–Lybrand.

Soothill, K. (1997) 'Rapists under 14 in the News', *Howard Journal* 36 (4): 367–77.

Stanko, E. and Hobdell, K. (1993) 'Assault on Men: Masculinity and Male Victimization', *British Journal of Criminology* 33 (3): 400–15.

Stanko, E., Crisp, D. Hale, C. and Lucraft, H. (1997) *Counting the Costs: Estimating the Impact of Domestic Violence in the London Borough of Hackney*, London: Crime Concern.

Starcevic, A. (1995) 'Touchy Subject', *Police Review* 17 February, pp. 18–19.

—— (1993) *The Ungentle Touch*, unpublished MA dissertation, University of Leicester.

Stiglmayer, A. (1993) 'The Rapes in Bosnia Herzegovina' in *Mass Rape: the War Against Women in Bosnia Herzegovina*, London: University of Nebraska.

Temkin, J. (1987) *Rape and the Legal Process*, London: Sweet & Maxwell.

—— (1993) 'Sexual History Evidence – The Ravishment of Section 2', *Criminal Law Review* 1: 3–20.

—— (1996)'Doctors, Rape and Criminal Justice', *The Howard Journal* 35 (1): 1–20.

—— (1997a) 'A Singular Victory', *Guardian*, G2 supplement, 11 September.

—— (1997b) 'Plus Ça Change: Reporting Rape in the 1990s', *British Journal of Criminology* 37: 507–27.

Toolis, K. (1993) 'Police Story', *Guardian*, 6 February.

Trade Union Congress (1983) *Sexual Harassment at Work*, London: TUC.

—— (1981) *Black Workers' Charter*, London: TUC.

Travis, A. (1998) 'Analysis: How to be a Judge', *Guardian*, 25 February.

UN Fourth World Conference on Women in Beijing (1995) *The Declaration and Platform for Action*, Beijing.

Utting, Sir William (1997) *Report of Tribunal Enquiry into Failings in Residential Care in North Wales*, London: Home Office.

Victim Support (1987) *Supporting Female Victims Of Sexual Assault: Training Manual*, London.

—— (1996) *Women, Rape and the Criminal Justice System*, London: Victim Support National Office.

Walklate, S. (1996) 'Equal Opportunities and the Future of Policing' in F. Leishman, B. Loveday and S.P. Savage (eds) *Core Issues in Policing*, London: Longman, pp. 191–204.

Walmsley, R. and White, K. (1979) *Sexual Offences, Consent and Sentencing*, Home Office Research Study No. 54, London: HMSO.

Weale, S. (1995) 'Private Case brings Rapist to Justice', *Guardian*, 18 May.

Weeks, J. (1977/1983) *Coming Out: Homosexual Politics from the19th Century to the Present*, London: Quartet Books.

Whittaker, B. (1979) *The Police in Society*, London: Eyre Methuen.

Williams, J.E. and Holmes, K.A. (1981) *The Sexual Assault*, Connecticut: Greenwood Press.

Williams, L. (1984) 'The Classic Rape: When do Victims Report?', *Social Problems* 31 (4).

Williamson, T. (1996) 'Police Investigation: The Changing Criminal Justice Context' in F. Leisham, B. Loveday and S.P. Savage (eds), *Core Issues in Policing*, London: Longman, pp. 26–38.

Wolmar, C. (1990) 'Police Are Advised To Give Higher Priority To Violence in Home', *Observer*, 1 August.

Women Against Rape and Legal Action for Women (1995) *Dossier: The Crown Prosecution Service and the Crime of Rape*, London: Crossroads.

Women's National Commission (1985) *Violence Against Women, Report of an Adhoc Working Group*, London: Cabinet Office.

*World in Action* (1989) 'The Right to Rape', ITV, 25 September.

—— (1997) 'Conduct Unbecoming', ITV, 20 October.

Wriggins, J. (1983) 'Rape, Racism and the Law', *Harvard Women's Law Journal* 6: 103–41.

Wright, R. (1984) 'A Note on Attrition of Rape Cases', *British Journal of Criminology* 24 (4): 399–400.

# Index